Overdue

ASH SUSPENSE THRILLERS
WITH A DASH OF ROMANCE
VOLUME IV

A Thriller

USA Today
Bestselling Author

Uvi Poznansky

Overdue@2021 Uvi Poznansky

All rights Reserved. No part of this book may be used or reproduced in any form or by any electronic or mechanical means, including information storage and retrieval system, without the written permission of the publisher, except by a reviewer who may quote brief passages in a review.

This is a work of fiction. Characters, names, places, and incidents are either the product of the author's imagination or are used fictitiously, and any resemblance to actual persons, living or dead, business establishments, locales, or events is entirely coincidental.

This novel can be read as a standalone novel, as well as a part of *Ash Suspense Thrillers with a Dash of Romance*.

Published by Uviart
P.O. Box 3233 Santa Monica CA 90408
Blog: uviart.blogspot.com
Email: uvi.author@gmail.com

First Edition 2021
Printed in the United States of America
Book design, cover image and cover design
Uvi Poznansky

Contents

Chapter 1 1
Chapter 2 12
Chapter 3 20
Chapter 4 28
Chapter 5 37
Chapter 6 46
Chapter 7 53
Chapter 8 59
Chapter 9 69
Chapter 10 78
Chapter 11 86
Chapter 12 94
Chapter 13 105
Chapter 14 112
Chapter 15 120
Chapter 16 128
Chapter 17 136
Chapter 18 144
Chapter 19 153
Chapter 20 161
Chapter 21 175
Chapter 22 184
Chapter 23 193
Chapter 24 200
About this Book 211
About the Author 212
About the Cover 215
Acknowledgments 217
A Note to the Reader 218

Bonus Excerpts 219
Books by Uviart 232

Chapter 1

One way for Vlad to avoid me, avoid paying the price for his crimes, is to play dead; another is to play dying. And who knows, perhaps it's for real. Perhaps it's not a game.

Still, I can't help but remain on guard, even if to others, it may seem pointless. Last time I saw him—about half a year ago—he lay contorted on the stretched hospital sheet, seemingly immobile, and never once lifted an eyelid to meet my gaze, which brought pity to my heart—but didn't expunge the fear.

I keep telling myself there's no reason anymore to be cautious. I shot him, and now he's said to be in a coma. About that, I have my doubts. Having spent enough time in his company before the hit, I know him all too well. Vlad rejoices in the pain he inflicts. To him, it means being in charge. He is not likely to relinquish it. Even if his power slips away, it's not going to be for long.

My brush with his Russian gang is something I'd like to forget. It left me struggling to piece my life together. Like an ink stain, the memory of what happened to me in their hands is somewhat shapeless and yet—indelible. Perhaps the only thing I can do now is give it more definition. If only I can learn his secrets.

I try to think the way he does. What would Vlad do now that the police arrested most of his gang, now that he is no longer in control? He would bide his time until finding the right moment to grab it again. And what better place to lay low than a hospital bed?

My boyfriend, Michael, says I'm overly suspicious. There's no way to fake being in a coma. I do want to believe that—but having been diagnosed a few months ago as a vegetable myself, I know from experience that faking it is not entirely out of the question. Especially when you start to regain your senses, and no one but you knows you're already alert.

So I just smile at him and say, "Time will tell."

Then, we move on to other subjects such as my job search, which unfortunately is next to impossible during the pandemic. Since my recent move to LA, I've been living out of my secondhand Ford Escape. This is merely a temporary measure, meant to reduce my expenses until I get hired. But these days, the job situation looks increasingly dire. *Temporary* is a tricky term. Who knows how long it can turn out to be?

Michael has been begging me to stay in Irvine with him for a few months, at least until a vaccine is developed, until it becomes widely available and the pandemic is over. I'm so tempted, not only because being together will make my life so much easier but also because when we're apart, I miss him.

Ma doesn't approve of Michael. For me, that adds a naughty allure to his proposition. She hates that he dropped out of college. In her eyes that's a sin, even if he committed it to start his own software company. On the other hand, she worries about me living by myself in an unsafe place. So she will definitely understand if I accept his offer.

Even so, I haven't. Blame my resistance on wanting to make something of myself. Blame it on being stubborn.

Michael is a software engineer who works out of his own garage. His most recent project is nothing short of fascinating. He has fused several types of scans from a real patient to create a view of the brain, which doctors can manipulate in virtual reality from multiple perspectives. The experience feels a bit like flying through a detailed, lifelike organ.

"Michael," I say, "what does a comatose brain look like?"

"Please, not that again." Michael drops his head into his hands. "You're totally obsessed with that Vlad."

"I do owe him a visit. It's long overdue—"

"Sweetheart, you owe nothing to that creep."

"You're right. I owe it to myself and to others, too, which I realize whenever I hear stories about survivors like me, struggling to find their way back to normal."

For a moment, Michael is silent.

"All right, Ash, I get it," he says at last. "I'll contact the hospital and check on him for you. And next time you come to Irvine, we'll go see him together."

"Thank you, Michael." I blink away tears. "It may be my last chance to ask him what I need to know; his last chance to confess. But I doubt he will."

*

That evening, we jog together along the slope, heading to Point Dume. Michael says the air will do me good.

His footfalls, fast and steady, soften when we reach the sand. As I turn to him, he extends his hand and touches mine. His smile, unmasked, reminds me that we're taking a risk. Given the rising death count, the state now mandates face covering—but at this remote location, who'll punish us for defying orders? Who'll condemn us for contaminating the air, for posing risk to others?

We stop and, hearts pounding, kiss.

His touch is sweet, his embrace—gentle. I'm tempted to lose myself in him, but can't let go of me. My eyes open even before he eases away.

Dark clouds are brushing the sky copper, their fiery edges sketched in reflection across the vast surface of water. After years of drought, an abundance of wildflowers has burst over the shoulder of the bluff, painting it mustard yellow. Tickseed flowers shake their toothed-tip petals, their scent sweetening the salty breeze.

Holding hands, we cross the line between the wind-blown dry sand and the wet, saturated seaboard. The beach looks different than I've expected. The cove, located just south of the Pointe, used to be famous as a popular clothing-optional meeting place back in the sixties, according to Ma. "Did your father ever mention where we first met? No?" She would snuff out the little smile flickering in the wrinkled corners of her lips. "Oh, the stories I could tell!"

But now, the place seems devoid of life. No clutter. No coolers, umbrellas, shade tents, barbecues or chairs. No one is sunbathing, with or without clothing. The place is deserted, not only because the air is bitterly cold this evening—which gives me sudden goosebumps—but also because of the latest prohibitions, meant to protect public health.

The sign says,

Keep it moving

Walking, surfing, and swimming are allowed—idle sitting is not.
Maintain a six-foot distance from others.
Use a hand sanitizer.
Pack out your trash.
Take it away with you

I rise to my tiptoes and slip my hands over Michael's shoulders, then run my fingers through his tousled hair, which is when I catch sight—just behind him—of something that begins to stir.

Squinting, I fix my eyes on it, which makes Michael take note. A seagull screeches past us, its chilling cry fluttering away over the water. A yawning wave breaks ashore. It spits a barefoot, flat-chested body onto the wet sand.

At first I think it's a man. The head is bald, or else shaven. The dark pants, tightly wrung around the legs, cling to the narrow hips. The white shirt, wrapped by algae, sticks to the ribs. The sleeves are dripping profusely as her fingers clutch at thin air.

She rises for a second and stumbles awkwardly, only to collapse—with barely a gasp—into my arms.

Her mouth opens.

No words come out.

I hear myself asking, "You all right?" and wish I could take the words back. The answer is clear. She's not.

The thought that she may be infected—that she may infect us—passes through my mind, but I set it aside. Social distancing? Forget it. Not now.

"Here," I say. "Let me give you a hand—"

Her knees buckle when I try to lift her, so Michael steps forward and catches her in his arms. She mumbles something that sounds a bit like *Voola,* but when I ask who or what it is, she narrows her eyes. Perhaps she's just too faint to keep them open.

"You need to see a doctor," he says. "Can we help you get there?"

She shakes her head, giving a long, incoherent moan.

"Where d'you live?"

"*Voola.*"

There it is again, that incomprehensible word.

Michael carries her along the shoreline as we head back to his Tesla. With each step, he gives a little grunt under her weight. His muscles glisten under the damp T-shirt. The only thing that makes him look like a nerd is his heavy, dark-rimmed glasses. He stops for a minute to push them up his nose.

Head lolling over his right shoulder, her eyelids droop over sunken cheeks. Knee over his left elbow, her foot dangles in the air, which draws my attention to a trickle of blood. It oozes out of a puncture hole in her heel, then slinks around it and drops off, afloat for just a second over the sea foam sloshing around us.

The wound goes on dripping along our way. For a while, we can't figure out what caused it—until I turn back and follow the trail of blood to its beginning. There, on the bank where we've found her, I spot something half-buried. Its tip catches the last ray of light.

"What did you find?" Michael asks, when I catch up with him.

"A discarded injection needle."

"Oh?"

"Probably used by some drug addict."

"She must have stepped on it, accidentally."

Is that what really happened? Where did she leave her shoes? Shall I ask her?

In her state, all she's going to say is *voola*.

Again, Michael stops for a breath. He lowers her and washes the sand off her injured foot. The sea water must hurt like hell—the poor woman comes out of her stupor in a big hurry to cry bloody murder—but then, what choice do we have? There is no fresh water anywhere in sight to cleanse the wound.

I take off my shirt, rip it in two, and tell Michael to stop staring at me. While he pretends to look away, I use one shred to apply pressure on her wound and bandage it.

He raises the woman. Step by step, they turn together to the parking lot, this time without leaving a trail of blood.

Meanwhile, I run back to pick up the needle. I wrap it in the remaining shred of my shirt, careful not to leave my own fingerprints, so I can hand it over to the police. How am I to know that I am being watched, and that this will set off a dangerous chain of events?

*

A week or so later, I get a FaceTime call from a long-time friend, Rita Caplan. Onscreen, she smacks her red lips together into a lovely smile. She must have just applied her makeup, a routine she admits is getting considerably more time-consuming at her late thirties, but she has never been one to shy away from vanity.

During the endless furlough from her sales job, Rita writes feel-good articles for an online magazine called *Malibu Daily*.

Her topics include the boom in property sales, as folks try to get away from the spread of the disease in the inner city; the success of fundraising for Malibu schools, as parents pray with waning hope for their safe reopening; and the comeback of drive-in movies, as everyone's attempt to avoid close contacts with others combines with the urge to escape reality.

Beyond writing fluff, Rita has grand aspirations. She's just unsure if she wants to become a writer of fiction, for which she has a way with words, or a TV reporter, for which she has an eye-catching pair of boobs. Either way, her best asset—which is annoying at times—is a curious mind.

Her eyes, blue-green like mine, shoot a sharp look at me. "I hear you're falling into a dangerous habit."

"What's that?"

"Getting in trouble."

Story of my life. I decide to take it as a joke, even though it's not all that funny. "What can I do? Wherever I go, it finds me."

"Seriously, Ash," she says. "You know what I'm talking about?"

Clueless, I shrug. "No, not really."

"That woman—"

"Which woman?"

"The one you called an ambulance for, a few days ago. I'm always eager for a good story, so no point keeping it a secret."

"Oh, yeah, Rita. I meant to tell you about her."

The scene surfaces back to mind, especially the part when the woman started coughing next to me in Michael's car and was barely able to catch her breath between one bout of wheezing and another.

It was at that moment that I stopped congratulating myself for rescuing her and instead, started to panic. Nowadays, germs are nothing to sneeze at.

Michael brought the car to an abrupt halt, and I jumped out of it even before he did. In my haste, I left my purse behind, next to her.

He placed a frantic 911 call, and an ambulance soon arrived. After the medics picked her up, we put on our masks, got back into the car, and—despite the daunting feeling of trepidation—worked furiously all evening to wipe every surface clean, as if our lives depended on it.

Correction: strike out *as if*.

Rita rolls her eyes. "How about, tell me what you know?"

"Besides being injured, that woman seemed terribly sick," I say. "Unfortunately, we didn't realize it at first. Do you know how is she now?"

"She was checked into UCLA," Rita says, "and less than an hour later—poof!—she vanished."

"What? How could she? I thought she was just about to draw her last breath—"

Rita shakes her head. "They took her temperature, administered some drugs, wrote down her information, and left her in a wheelchair, until they could arrange for a makeshift ICU bed. Somehow, when no one was looking, she managed to take off."

"I don't believe it! Can anyone at the hospital explain how this could happen?"

"No."

"No?"

"Trust me, I asked. UCLA is swamped with cases. The fact that a patient disappears is an embarrassment—but life goes on. Death goes on too, the sick keep coming in, bodies keep piling up... The medical staff must move on, must try to save the next patient."

I throw my hands up in the air, and Rita asks, "D'you happen to know the name of that woman?"

"No, I don't—"

"Too bad. She used yours."

I swallow the first thing that comes to mind—*Ha?*—and instead mutter, "Excuse me?"

"She used your driver's license," says Rita, this time in a deliberately measured manner, as if explaining an overly complex problem to someone slow to understand. "And, she used your medical insurance."

For a second, I'm speechless. It's a good thing I have a chair behind me, because my knees give out.

All week, I assumed that once everything falls into place, I would manage, somehow, to find these documents. Their strange disappearance annoyed me. While in a self-imposed quarantine, I emptied my purse time and again, turned every pocket inside out, traced back my actions. Keep calm, I told myself. No need to lose sleep over nothing, right?

But lose sleep I did. I couldn't avoid thinking, with a scowl on my face much like Ma's, that no one is to blame for this loss but me, because my life falls, all too often, into chaos. And whose fault is that? How could I be so disorganized?

The notion that my driver license as well as my medical insurance card got stolen did occur to me—but I laughed it off. The last thing I feared was identity theft.

"It gets worse," Rita says. "Thanks to that woman, your medical record in the UCLA system has been updated."

"What?" I cry. "How?"

"Now, it states you are a heroin addict."

"I'm not—"

"But she is!"

I say nothing for a long while, so Rita presses on. "Quite conveniently, that woman presented herself as you, Ash. And from now on—if not caught in the act—she'll continue to do so."

I shake my head, still in utter disbelief.

"Rita," I say, at last, "I found a heroin needle not far from where we found her and then, later that same night, turned it over to the police."

"Oh really?"

"Really."

"They must have some DNA results by now," she says, her voice perking up. "I have my connections, you know? Perhaps I can help."

"Will you?"

"I'll let you know what I find."

Chapter 2

Dreary moments tick past midnight. I open the sunroof of my clunker a crack to bring in some air. Hours later, I remain sleepless. Stars begin to fade. My mood darkens.

It's been a week since I talked with Rita and since I asked the police to investigate the case of my stolen identity. I suppose they have their hands full with more pressing stuff these days—but what excuse does Rita have for not getting back to me?

I wonder, has her police friend agreed to help? Has he succeeded in tracking down the DNA results from the heroin needle I found? Do these results belong to the woman who stole my identity? What's her real name? Was she truly sick? Was she contagious?

If her excessive coughing was merely an act, *Ms. Voola* need not worry about her health like the rest of us, because I'm going to kill her. She must be punished for making a hermit out of me. Thanks to her, I've self-quarantined until today, and so has Michael.

Now, I hear a knock and his voice, calling my name.

Bolting out of the Escape with a slam of the door, "Nothing," I say, when Michael asks what's wrong. His hand is still raised in the air for a second knock as I walk past him.

My body is stiff from tossing and turning for hours. I bought the secondhand Ford Escape for less than five thousand bucks—

nearly my entire savings at the time—removed the back seats, built a bed frame out of two-by-twos, secured it in place, fixed a carpeted plywood sheet on top, and covered it with a few foam sections. The sleeping platform allows enough room for both my dog Browny and me. I'm proud of my handiwork, but falling asleep on it? Somehow, that's hard.

Michael wears a crisp shirt, lose-fitting jeans, and two-days' growth of bristles fighting hard to get through the skin and make him look rugged. Never saw him this way before. So handsome.

Without another word, he weaves his fingers into mine. The joy of feeling him gives me a little jolt—but then, so does the envy. Unlike me, he has the luxury of sleeping in a regular bed.

"I know how you feel, sweetheart. The isolation we've had to endure these last two weeks is driving me crazy, too," Michael says. "I can't help thinking about what it's doing to us."

"For you," I say, my tone irate, "it can't be all that difficult, being safe at home, earning good money out of what you do best, those virtual simulations of yours."

"Got bored with *safe*, sweetheart."

"Still, it's easy for you, having a glorious good time with those software games—"

"Got bored with *easy*."

I look away, saying nothing.

Michael turns my chin with a finger and looks deep and long into my eyes. "I don't know about you, but shutting myself away makes me moody."

Moody is just where I am, just where I want to stay. Stubborn, that's me. So I go on saying nothing.

Michael cups my face with his hands. "Oh, Ash, when I noticed your location on the GPS, I realized that the middle of nowhere is no place for you to spend the night. So, I drove all the way over—"

"For what?" I step away from his touch. "To save me?"

"Yes, Ash, and me, too—"

"I may be a damsel in distress, but I can save myself from it."

"You sure?"

"Sure I'm sure!"

"All right then, sweetheart." He bends over my Golden Retriever, sinks his fingers in the fluffy fur, and rubs him fondly between the ears till Browny's eyes close to a slit. "I suppose," Michael says, "this isn't the right time to ask you something sensitive?"

"Such as what?"

He dashes forward, opens his arms with flair, and kneels down smack in front of me. "Such as, will you marry me?"

I pull back. "No. It isn't."

Without losing a beat, he hops back to his feet. "I wasn't going to."

Michael turns away, scanning the mountain view as if in search for a roundabout way to reach the reasonable side of me.

Fooled him! There isn't any.

I pace to and fro, Browny trotting after me. The beauty of the landscape—marred by the Woolsey Fire damage of a few years ago and the neglect of recent months—shines in the darkness all around us every now and again, as the moon peeks out from the trees. Its faint rays flicker on the jagged edges of broken bottles strewn along the horseshoe bend of the road. If not for this light, I may lose a step.

Using his remote, Michael turns on the headlights of his Tesla. A large stone sign, partially swallowed by a thick overgrowth, glistens out of the shadows. On it, a crack zigzags through the engraved *Charmlee Wilderness Park*.

As a child, I used to visit this place with my parents. At that time, they were still together. Coming here, I hoped to revive happy memories—only to learn that the park has been closed. In these troubled times, who knows when it'll reopen.

Nothing stays the same.

Michael matches his step to mine and takes my hand. "I suppose it isn't the right time for this other thing, too, but I'm going to do it anyway."

"No," I mutter. "It isn't—"

"Don't be so sure, sweetheart." He pulls me into the shadows, away from the bright headlights, and wraps his fingers around my neck. His hand is firm. It makes my skin tingle.

"No," I repeat, but this time with little conviction. Then, I hear myself whispering, "Maybe."

Michael brings me to his heart and gives me a kiss. Sweet at first. Then, different. Passionate.

And in a snap—poof!—the blackness that weighed me down is gone. It's not sunrise yet, but my day begins to brighten.

In his embrace, I'm home.

We cling to each other. "Kiss me, Michael," I murmur in his ear.

It's not just my tone, softening. I practically melt in his arms. I'm in heat. I bet he feels it, too. In his naughty voice, he says, "Wait. I have a little something for you."

"Do you?"

"I do," he says. "From your Ma."

*

At the first signs of outbreak, the spring semester at UCI ended abruptly, which drove me away from campus in search of a job. With all those cutting-edge engineering courses under my belt, as well as some experience designing virtual reality gadgets for my boyfriend, I thought landing an offer would be a piece of cake. Well, it wasn't. Then, I figured that if all else fails, I could make do for a while as a hairdresser or a waitress. How hard can that be? Customers can be forgiving. And generous, too. I'll get paid even for the mistakes I make.

But so far, tough luck. Restaurants have closed, and so have beauty parlors.

With a little kvetch, Ma accepted my move from Irvine to Los Angeles, where—with a bit of good fortune—more opportunities may be found. As I drove away, she waved goodbye to me out of her kitchen window, eyes tearful, lips pursed.

My heart aches, even now, to think how afraid she must have been—afraid for me to go and afraid for me to stay. Pa, who stood there behind her, tried to grin. His smile, such as it was, wore doubt. Unlike any time in the past, he held back his advice. Perhaps he had none, because who knows what's a safe place these days. Everywhere you go, an aggressively spreading virus can reach out for you.

They accepted my move, but disapproved of my decision not to rent a place. For me, that decision was easy. Sleeping in an

SUV is the new norm nowadays for young people out of work, a new way of being resourceful. The hard part is learning how to manage on the road. Armed with a list of all legal overnight parking spots in Los Angeles, I never park in the same spot two nights in a row.

Since my departure from the city where I grew up, my boyfriend has been filling in for me, taking care of my parents. Nothing he does will ever endear him to Ma—but for some reason, he persists. Every Friday, Michael delivers groceries to her doorstep, so she doesn't have to rub elbows with other shoppers. That's no fun lately, due to the all-too-real threat of infection.

"So." I pull at his sleeve. "What about that little something from Ma?"

Michael chuckles. "She called me late at night, saying she can't fall asleep, and she hopes I don't mind her calling me at this godless hour, and wouldn't I get there at once, because she's distraught, and so is your father, because of the food shortages and whatnot, and all that's left in her pantry is a bit of yeast and a nearly empty bag of flour, and who knows what'll happen next. I got to her place and—guess what?—found her in the middle of baking."

"Really?"

"Really. And—get this—she gave me two loaves of her wonderful homemade challah bread, steaming hot from the oven."

"Wow!"

"I told her I'll savor every morsel, and she said, 'Don't you get any funny ideas, young man. I still think you're wrong for Ashley.'"

Michael opens the passenger-side door of his Tesla and takes out a picnic basket. What's inside? A bottle of red wine, two wine glasses, napkins, and two loaves, beautifully braided, glazed with egg wash and sprinkled with sesame seed. Nestled inside a clean, carefully folded kitchen towel, they're still slightly warm to the touch.

We climb onto the sleeping platform inside my Escape. Browny tries to crawl into the dent between us, then gives up and curls on the driver's seat, his tail giving a flick against the driving wheel now and then. Through the open sunroof, Michael and I watch the first rays of sunrise, tickling the clouds with a hesitant touch of pink.

We eat. We drink. We snuggle.

And just as I'm about to say, "Don't get any funny ideas, young man," a sudden rattling noise makes me freeze.

Is it one of the choppers? The sky over Los Angeles has been crowded with them lately. Some belong to TV stations covering the unrest. Others are federal helicopters, monitoring the riots. A few have no markings whatsoever.

Michael sits up. "This noise, whatever it is, is not in the sky." His voice is low, but full of alarm. "Shhh... Listen. Something's coming up the road."

I peer out through the tinted side-window, hoping not to be noticed. An unidentified gray van rambles by, its driver glancing blankly in the direction of my secondhand clunker, before stopping on the opposite side of the road, next to Michael's shiny Tesla. Four figures—four men in unmarked camouflage wear, wide leather belts, and glassy face shields fixed to their military helmets—file out.

I duck down next to Michael, not before catching sight of them surrounding his car. By the sound of it, they're kicking its fancy tires with their boots. My heart drops a notch with each kick.

Who are they? Why are they here? What do they want?

Michael opens the liftgate of the Escape just enough to let him slip through. I crawl out after him. The moment we hit the ground, a stench of gasoline hits us, spreading in the air. It comes from the direction of his car, which is strange because the Tesla is all electric. Michael is so proud of his big toy, which he assembled with his own hands. It requires no oil changes, fuel filters, spark plug replacements or emission checks.

The men close in on the Tesla. What on earth are they doing? Admiring its innovative design? Its sleek lines? No, not really. One of them is holding a five-gallon rigid container by its angled handle. With each stride, he's pouring a dark liquid through the spout, aiming it at the car.

Michael lets out a groan, then grits his teeth. I've never seen him like this, fighting to hold back rage.

I don't want him to go, don't want him to confront them, whoever they are, even as they're marching back to the unmarked van. So I grab Michael hard, straining every muscle, every fiber in me. But before I can say a word—*whoomph*—the Tesla ignites, licked by flames.

Chapter 3

The blaze consuming the Tesla with a hungry roar is so bright, so utterly spectacular that I stare at it, mesmerized. I forget to run away. Michael grabs hold of Browny and pulls both of us into a ditch. I lie flat by his side, panting, under a shower of sparks. Debris rains from the sky, landing all around.

Opposite us, the four men in camouflage don't seem to notice our presence. At first, I fear they'll set fire to my Escape as well, just for grins. To my surprise, they simply ignore it—all but one. He glances at it, then waves a hand in dismissal as if to say, *Forget it. Not my job.* Turning their backs to the clunker, they pat each other's shoulders, a camaraderie of evil celebrated at our expense.

The leader of the pack gives a thumbs-up as the other three climb into the unidentified van. He lowers the driver side window, takes the wheel and, while making a U-turn, smiles broadly at his handiwork, the burning thing that used to be a Tesla. The tires have begun to melt, smoldering on one side. Black, acrid smoke is beginning to reach us. Soon, it'll be hard to breathe.

As the van passes by the ditch, the man says something to the other three—it sounds, oh, I don't know, like *Voola?*—and they burst into loud, rolling laughter. Which is a good thing, because it covers up my dry croak.

Have they noticed it?

My teeth are chattering uncontrollably. The sound is maddening to me. Have they caught it? Will they come back for us?

No. The van rambles down the road and turns around the bend. A moment later, it's gone.

Are we safe?

I raise my head. The flames soar overhead, licking higher and higher into the night sky. Billowing smoke starts to thicken around us. It drifts over the trees and across the road, creating an intermittent view of the mountains. The wind picks up and feeds the fire.

Blowing in my face is a wave of heat. In spite of it, I shiver. "W—why—what was that all about?"

Michael rises to his feet and gives me a hand. His chin is set, his face—pale. "That," he says, darkly, "was a warning."

*

What does that mean, *a warning*? Against doing what? Who's behind it? And why?

No time to ask. Sparks fly overhead like it's a regular Fourth of July. Tongues of fire curl here and there around us, exploring the ground, hissing, hesitating slightly, licking embers here and there, then slithering towards the Escape.

As I run to the car, smoke erupts, clouding my vision. Overcome by it, Browny has stopped barking. I take him in my arms. The only thing that guides me through as I fumble forward is Michael's voice. "Can you see me?"

"No," I cry. "Where are you?"

"Over here, next to the passenger side of your car," he says. "Careful now—"

In a blink, I bump against a tire. My hand scrabbles desperately across some surface, fingers grazing every curve, every dent, even though the metal is scorching to the touch. Oh, it's a door. I find the handle blindly, tear it open, and let Browny in. Then I leap onto the driver seat.

My hands sweat as I insert the key into the ignition. "C'mom, c'mon," I say, but the car refuses to start.

Michael buckles up. He must be holding himself back from saying, "Damn! I told you not to buy this piece of junk."

"Oh no," I stammer, heatedly slapping the steering wheel. "C'mon already!"

Nothing.

I take the key out, stick it back in, twist, then again. Oh boy. It's going to be a long way home.

Especially if we have to walk.

Then, the engine emits a cough, then a few more sporadic whirring noises just for good measure. At last—oh, it's running!

Meanwhile, Michael calls 911 and reports a case of arson to the authorities. He tells them that his vehicle was set on fire and asks them to send firefighters right away, so the blaze doesn't spread and cause more damage than it already did.

Accelerating up the road, I drive away from the intensifying flames. In the rearview mirror, I see them wrapping over the trees behind us, engulfing them.

"Where to?" I ask.

And Michael says, "My place."

I give him a reluctant look. "It's rush hour."

"I know how tired you are." He leans over and gives me a little peck. "Would you like me to take the wheel?"

"No." I roll my eyes. "Still, it's a two-hour drive. Maybe more."

"Maybe less. There should be no traffic because of the Stay-at-Home order—"

"Ah, it was issued a month ago. By now, people are sick of it."

Michael shakes his head. "If they don't obey it, they'll be sick for real."

He seems to need a smile. I give it to him. "Your place, then?"

"Yes, sweetheart. I want you to see something."

"How about a little hint?"

"What happened to my Tesla is merely a warning. There's more to come."

I peer out the window as a siren starts shrieking in the distance. A strobing of red and white emergency lights marks a procession of in-coming fire engines.

I wait for him to explain his cryptic remark, but Michael seems too upset to talk. His face is stern. Finally he says, "If anything happens to me, you must know what I learned about a particular friend of yours."

✲

The garage door closes with a whoosh behind us. We're inside, at last. Two hours ago, back at the gas station, I disabled my cellphone's GPS tracking system and so did Michael, so no one could follow us. We're safe. Or so we think.

The garage sets me at ease, usually. It's where Michael created his virtual reality startup, before selling it off to a military ops company. At the time, he asked me to design gadgets such as VR gloves. Working together was fun. We developed not only games but also training programs for the food industry. We made it possible for their employees to interact remotely with their virtual job surroundings and learn the required tasks, such as dealing with Walmart's holiday rush or mastering the espresso pull.

I can't help but think that engineering the future seems laughable now, because the present is dramatically different from how we imagined it would be. What we would call *post-apocalyptic* back then turns out to be the new reality.

Because of the virus, people won't even set foot in restaurants. Michael's previous neighbor used to be a well-paid manager at the casual-fare restaurant chain, California Pizza Kitchen, before it filed for bankruptcy. His voice rings loud and clear next to the garbage cans. He's rummaging for food, trying to fight off other homeless drifters.

I plop down in the corner of the garage. Its walls are painted blue so they can disappear into the background when Michael conjures his simulated virtual environment. Normally, I relax into this dreamy atmosphere, but not now. My heart is pounding too hard.

It's a relief, almost, to feel it skipping a beat when my cellphone rings. "Rita! Any news?"

"None too good," she says, a bit uneasily. "Let me ask, did you happen to cash the savings in your account?"

"No, I didn't—"

"Well, Ash, someone did it for you."

"What?" I say, hearing my voice rising to a pitch. "And how would you even know that?"

"How else? Through my police friend," says Rita. "Yesterday, he was dispatched to the Malibu branch of Wells Fargo bank. According to his report, their security system was compromised."

"What about my money?"

"You're on their surveillance video, stashing bills into a duffle bag."

"B-but," I stammer, "but that can't be!"

"My friend matched the face to what's available on record on you."

"Then, he made a mistake."

"A face recognition algorithm was used—"

"Every algorithm," says Michael, cutting in, "can be fooled."

I ask, "Was the imposter wearing face covering?"

"Good question," says Rita. "I don't know."

"Can you get your hands on that video?"

"I doubt it, but I'll try." She waves her hand in parting and smiles. "Have to run. Talk soon—"

"Wait!" I jump to my feet, as if I could chase her from afar. "I thought you're calling about something else, about the DNA traces on that needle—"

"Working on it, Ash." In the manner of TV anchors, which she mimics so perfectly, Rita teases, "Stay tuned," and ends the call.

*

For a moment, I stare into thin air, lost in utter confusion. Instead of getting some clarity from her, Rita has given me one more riddle to solve. My identity was ripped off, my money—stolen.

What a bummer.

Bummer is too weak a word, considering what I feel. I'm tempted to mutter something more crude, more explicit—something you can't say in polite company.

On second thought, here it is. Fuck.

Michael raises an eyebrow as if he can hear my thoughts. Then he heads for the kitchen. "Hungry?"

I follow, then put on an apron. "I am!"

In a small bowl, Michael whisks together eggs, milk, and vanilla. He swirls in a pinch of cinnamon, a dash of nutmeg, and a bit of sugar, then pours the mixture into a pie plate.

Meanwhile, I melt butter in a skillet, swooning over the gentle aroma. Boy, *hungry* is not the right word for what I feel. *Famished* is more like it.

Michael cuts the remainder of my mother's challah bread into thick slices. He dips each slice in turn in the batter and fries one side to golden brown perfection. In one smooth movement, he flips it high in the air—perhaps trying to impress me—and lets it land with a splat onto the spatula.

Once the other side is fried, I remove the masterpiece from the skillet, set it on a plate with a few fresh strawberries, and drizzle maple syrup on top.

We gobble down one French toast after another. We lick the plate clean. He licks my fingers. We kiss.

Aroused, I nibble at his ear. I whisper, "What now?"

"What?" I say, hearing my voice rising to a pitch. "And how would you even know that?"

"How else? Through my police friend," says Rita. "Yesterday, he was dispatched to the Malibu branch of Wells Fargo bank. According to his report, their security system was compromised."

"What about my money?"

"You're on their surveillance video, stashing bills into a duffle bag."

"B-but," I stammer, "but that can't be!"

"My friend matched the face to what's available on record on you."

"Then, he made a mistake."

"A face recognition algorithm was used—"

"Every algorithm," says Michael, cutting in, "can be fooled."

I ask, "Was the imposter wearing face covering?"

"Good question," says Rita. "I don't know."

"Can you get your hands on that video?"

"I doubt it, but I'll try." She waves her hand in parting and smiles. "Have to run. Talk soon—"

"Wait!" I jump to my feet, as if I could chase her from afar. "I thought you're calling about something else, about the DNA traces on that needle—"

"Working on it, Ash." In the manner of TV anchors, which she mimics so perfectly, Rita teases, "Stay tuned," and ends the call.

∗

For a moment, I stare into thin air, lost in utter confusion. Instead of getting some clarity from her, Rita has given me one more riddle to solve. My identity was ripped off, my money—stolen.

What a bummer.

Bummer is too weak a word, considering what I feel. I'm tempted to mutter something more crude, more explicit—something you can't say in polite company.

On second thought, here it is. Fuck.

Michael raises an eyebrow as if he can hear my thoughts. Then he heads for the kitchen. "Hungry?"

I follow, then put on an apron. "I am!"

In a small bowl, Michael whisks together eggs, milk, and vanilla. He swirls in a pinch of cinnamon, a dash of nutmeg, and a bit of sugar, then pours the mixture into a pie plate.

Meanwhile, I melt butter in a skillet, swooning over the gentle aroma. Boy, *hungry* is not the right word for what I feel. *Famished* is more like it.

Michael cuts the remainder of my mother's challah bread into thick slices. He dips each slice in turn in the batter and fries one side to golden brown perfection. In one smooth movement, he flips it high in the air—perhaps trying to impress me—and lets it land with a splat onto the spatula.

Once the other side is fried, I remove the masterpiece from the skillet, set it on a plate with a few fresh strawberries, and drizzle maple syrup on top.

We gobble down one French toast after another. We lick the plate clean. He licks my fingers. We kiss.

Aroused, I nibble at his ear. I whisper, "What now?"

"Not what you think." Michael slips out of my arms and off his seat. Then, he brings in two VR headsets.

"So?" he says. "You ready for trouble?"

I follow him to the garage. "Ready I am!"

Only now do I understand why we came here, of all places. Seeking safety, which can be illusive, was only a minor part of the reason. The more crucial part was finding a way to figure out that inexplicable warning, that threat that cost Michael his car.

What better place than his garage, where virtual realities that spring from his computer can be played out in full scale? Where else can we step into remote locations and study them up close?

"So." I put on my VR headset. "What's the plan?"

Michael enters a key sequence into his laptop. "I'm going to show you where I went after our last date, and what I discovered."

"Give me a clue, will you?"

"Someone must have noticed me poking around. He had me followed. His men destroyed my Tesla—but spared me. For now."

"I think I know who it is—"

"I hope you do, Ash. And I hope you understand the way he thinks, because my life may depend on it."

"Vlad?"

"We're going to pay him a visit."

"Really?"

"Virtually."

"Even so," I say, "it's long overdue."

Chapter 4

There's a good reason why it's taken me that long to go see Vlad. I'd rather do something else, anything, because the prospect of spending time in that man's company gives me the creeps.

Michael slings his arm across my shoulders and gives me a gentle squeeze. "You all right?"

I shrug.

He takes off his VR headset and gives me a worried look.

"I'm fine, just fine," I say, feeling anything but.

And as soon as these words part my lips, bad memories flash across my mind.

The first time I met Vlad was when I turned fourteen. I came to see Pa at work and found Vlad sitting in his chair. He took over my father's job at Southern California Edison. Because of the way he ogled me, I sensed that he was trouble—and not only for my father.

The feeling was vague. Back then, no one I knew had any idea about his shady past in the KGB or his even shadier role in organized crime. Only now do I begin to recognize his fingerprints in multiple muddy projects, from the shutoff of the electrical grid in the entire state of California to large-scale health insurance fraud to child sex trafficking.

At the time, the notion that Vlad would be sending his thugs after me seemed laughable. How could I guess he was biding his time, waiting for the right moment to take me, calculating what he could demand in exchange for my freedom?

The second time he saw me I was in a coma, thanks to having been beaten senseless by one of the goons he sent to abduct me. That guy couldn't resist having a bit of fun on the side at my expense.

Lying on a hospital bed, I must have looked like a mummy, all wrapped up in bandages—but that didn't prevent Vlad from snatching me out of there and holding me hostage. He stashed me away in a dark hotel room in his suite while negotiating the ransom.

What was his risk in having me this close to him? None. No wonder Vlad let down his defenses. In his eyes, I was damaged goods. I was dead.

Well, almost.

Despite appearances to the contrary, my senses started to come back. First came smell. Then hearing. I could, somehow, capture every word uttered around me. So I got to know Vlad and his operation quite well. And I realized, with great dread, that I might not live to tell the tale.

In hindsight, treating me like a broken doll was his mistake. It cost him dearly. As a practical joke, his goon hung a pistol on my thumb just as I was struggling to regain some control over it. How could he miss the gleam in my eyes? It took everything I had in me to pull that trigger.

And then, when everyone least expected—*boom!*—a bullet flew out. Now, don't blame me for being a bad shot. Let's see how you aim when you're only half awake! The bullet missed the goon—but by a strange reversal of fortune, it knocked Vlad into a vegetative state.

Given my own brush with coma, I suspected Vlad could hear sounds even as he lay in the ICU bed, seemingly immobile. During my first visit, I could barely recognize him. His face, looking somewhat blurry under the clear plastic ventilator mask, was utterly contorted.

His mind wasn't something I wished to understand. To crawl into it would be sickening. Once there, I would find myself locked in a dark place. But I felt compelled to sit by his bedside and study him. There was little choice in the matter.

After all, I knew nothing about his goon, the one who violated me. I had no name for him, not even a face. All I could recall was his voice. I had to find him. He had to be punished. This was a must, not only to gain closure—if there is such a thing—but to protect other girls.

And Vlad could help, if he wanted to. He could tell me the thug's name, his habits, his hiding place. I had to keep my eyes on Vlad until he came to. I had to make him talk.

But then… Then came the plague.

At first, the hospital seemed emptier than usual. Visits to the ER dropped sharply. Family members were banned from accompanying ailing patients, except in special cases such as end-of-life. Somewhat reluctantly, the nurses let me in. They thought we were family—and in an awkward way, they were right. His life was tied with mine. The knot was painful.

Sitting by his bedside, I did something that might have astonished him. It surprised even me. I drew near Vlad and—

doing my best not to upset the IV tube attached to his wrist—took his hand in mine. The tips of his fingers were ice-cold.

"Here we meet again," I said.

Bringing to mind his perfect British accent, I half-expected him to use it, but no. A low, gurgling sound burbled from deep down in his throat.

I took it to mean, "Damn you! You are the reason I am here."

"Look, Vlad—"

The machines emitted a series of beeps, which I translated into a string of colorful expletives, some of them expressed in his native Russian, others in his Oxford English, followed by, "I can't even open my eyes, and it's all your fault. The hell with you, bitch! Get out!"

I pulled up a chair, made myself comfortable and, in my coolest, most businesslike tone, said, "Listen, Vlad. Coma is nothing to sneeze at. You're going to stay here a while. And whether you like it or not, I'll be keeping an eye on you."

Cutting me off was another gurgling sound.

"Oh stop it," I said. "Consider my presence a good thing, will you? As long as you have visitors, you aren't forgotten."

He puffed out a snore.

"You're going to grow tired of me," I promised. "I'll hound you constantly, even as you sleep. Unless—"

His eyeballs rolled in their sockets, showing all white.

"Unless," I stressed, "You give me what I want."

He blinked.

"Snap out of your sleep," I said, "just long enough to spill the truth."

Was he looking at me? I searched for any hint, any shade of expression that might be flitting across those pale blue eyes. Perhaps he felt the weight of my gaze. Perhaps he realized I couldn't be fooled. With me, he couldn't pretend to be absent.

He might have known what I wanted, but just in case he didn't, I spelled it out. "I'll go away and not bother you again, if you tell me the name of your thug. The one who disobeyed your orders and raped me."

Vlad fell completely silent. This time, there was not even a gurgling sound.

I hated to repeat myself, but felt compelled to do so. "What's his name?"

His blue lips clamped under the ventilator mask. Vlad was holding a secret.

I rose to my feet. "Where do I find him?"

Nothing. Not even a twitch.

Overcoming a revulsion, I stepped closer and smoothed the blanket over him. "You can help, Vlad. Sleep on it."

And on that note, I left.

Every week since then, I would call UCI Medical Center, and the nurses would tell me about his vital signs. According to them, the graphs flatlined, almost—which I didn't want to believe.

Was this some kind of a game? Was the Russian capable of slowing his own heart rate? Did he have an accomplice at the hospital, someone who could fiddle with the machine? Or was there a problem with its readout? Was my suspicion way overblown? Was Vlad truly on the verge of dying?

Michael tucks an unruly curl behind my ear while looking searchingly into my eyes. "Ash? You ready?"

I thread my fingers through his. "Sure. What's the worst that can happen?"

*

Michael adjusts the VR headset so it fits snugly over my eyes. He seems to know where we're going—but to me, the vision is confusing, at first. With a click of a key on his cellphone, he conjures up a corridor. Instantly, its 3D image fills the air, blurring blue garage walls into near oblivion.

"What is this?" I ask. "Where are we?"

Michael calibrates some controls, sharpening corners, bringing lines into focus so now the image looks less sketchy. At the same time, he raises an eyebrow. "Don't you know?"

"Oh yes, I do! UCI Medical Center."

"I had the opportunity to go there last week, because of an experimental project I'm working on for the hospital. So I thought I'd also drop in on our so-called friend."

I snort. "Vlad?"

"Exactly," says Michael. "I connected my cellphone to a miniature omnidirectional camera. You know the clunky little thing."

"I do."

"Through it, I streamed the recorded video data into my virtual reality model. So now, we can study the scene and everything I saw, at our leisure."

I take a step in one direction of the virtual corridor—only to correct myself and turn the other way. With every step, I have to keep reminding myself that nothing in this space is real. It is the memory of a visit, digitally stored.

Even the figures in nurse uniforms are apparitions, constructed from digital bytes and projected into position. Medics come and go around us, seemingly smiling, or that's how I read the shape of breath crimping their fabric masks: at times denting, at times puffing the fabric.

Walking a bit too fast, I pass though the ghost of one of them and find myself startled to see her falling apart into clumps, into pixels. No matter. Materializing again, she points at a door. It is swaying on its virtual hinges, slightly ajar.

I put on my VR glove. Its touch sensors will let me interact with the elements of this place not only by vision but also by feel. Then I push open the virtual door, relishing the sense of how heavy it is, how it resists giving way.

On its other side, next to an IV pole, is an ICU bed.

Empty.

Bathed in unreal sunlight that streams in through a window, the bed is bare. Its air mattress platform, designed for pressure relief, has been stripped off. Soiled bedsheets are draped over a hamper in the corner of the space. This virtual model hasn't yet been upgraded to include smell. Now that's a relief.

I touch the bed, feel its corner bumpers, its castors. Strangely, it seems to have been stopped in the middle of performing its innovative tilting process, known to help turn the patient gently, minimizing physical effort. The plastic side rails have been dropped. There are no readout graphs on the overhead screens. No blinking lights, no beeps.

Just an eerie silence.

"So? Where's Vlad?" I demand, doing my best to contain a growing sense of disappointment. "I thought we're about to see him."

"So did I," says Michael.

"What?"

"I was told he passed away quietly."

"No fair. He can't do that to me!"

Of all the possible things I feared might happen, this—to me—is the most dreadful. In my book, a criminal must meet his just punishment. How did Vlad manage to escape it? How brazen of him to die before telling me the name of his goon, the one who beat me senseless and who can now remain at large. The thug knows where Ma lives, so he can lay a trap for me there—but I have no clue about his whereabouts.

That's not how things were supposed to happen.

Greatly annoyed, I grab the cellphone from Michael and with a click, put an abrupt end to the phantom environment. "I drove us here all the way from LA after a sleepless night, for that?"

The hospital bed vanishes—*poof!*—into thin air, followed by the fluid med containers that hang from the IV pole, followed by the pole itself, followed by a last flash, shooting across a fading impression of its hooks.

Michael reaches for me. "Wait."

I slap the cellphone into his palm. "There's nothing to wait for, now."

"Ash, wait, there's more—"

"You don't get it, Michael, do you? I'm so angry. I can't even begin to tell you how angry I am."

"Sweetheart—"

"Don't you *sweetheart* me. How dare Vlad find a way out of my life without leaving me a hint of how I can put it back together?"

Michael tries to block my way, but my anguish makes me push him aside. I storm out of his garage and stomp across the street. The homeless, still probing through emptied garbage bags, glance at me from the corners of their eyes, as if to assess the threat I may pose to them.

Meanwhile, shots ring in the distance. I ignore them. Probably police forces sent to quell some riots.

Then, a single shot blasts out, this one at close range.

I run back to Michael just as he begins to collapse. My heart skips a beat as his head hits the blue cement floor, his shoulder smearing it red.

Chapter 5

Michael stirs, which gives me something I desperately need. Hope. Overcoming a quiver, I unbutton his shirt to ease his labored breathing, then stare at the wound just to the left of the base of his neck. It is surrounded by a reddish-brown ring of abraded skin. Lodged above his collar bone, barely seen through a thin film of blood, is a metallic thing. A bullet. Not something I can handle on my own, if his life is to be saved.

I cradle his head, lay it in my lap ever so gently, then remove the VR headset from his eyes.

Michael raises trembling fingers to his left shoulder. He does it slowly, with effort, as if fighting to find his way through a dizzy spell, through a fog that is closing in on him alone. Then, bringing his fingers to his eyes, he gazes in disbelief at the red smudge on their tips.

I pull my cellphone from the back pocket of my jeans and call 911.

Michael clutches my elbow and with heart-wrenching agony, croaks, "No. Don't—"

"I must, my love." My eyes well with tears.

I report the shooting and, even before I have the chance to specify Michael's address, I hear a siren. As if to answer my prayers, it comes closer, sharply searing the air.

"Never mind," I say to the 911 operator, "I hear the ambulance coming."

"Wait," says the operator. "We'll need to ask a few questions—"

"And I'll be happy to answer."

"We're sending a detective to talk to you—"

"Not now," I say. "Later."

With a startle, Michael grabs my hand. I bend over to kiss his. My tears stream down his chiseled cheekbone, making the stubble on his chin glisten. "Don't talk," I plead. "Help's coming. Any moment now."

"Sweet—"

"Shhh, babe."

"Sweetheart." His groan trembles in the cool morning air. "There's more."

Stroking his brow, I echo, "More?"

His head lolls between my thighs. He's not hearing me, is he?

"More?"

No answer.

Paramedics arrive. Three men with no skin exposed. One of them holds a remote—no, not a remote exactly, but a non-contact infrared thermometer which he aims at Michael, at his temple. Then, he aims it at me. Judging by their sigh of relief, neither Michael nor I show signs of fever, which means we do not pose a threat of infection to them. Even so, they tell me to step aside while they dress Michael's wound and load him onto a stretcher.

"Will he live?" I ask, choked by tears.

Not really answering, they tell me to stay behind. I'm not allowed to accompany Michael to UCI Medical Center. Such are the regulations these days, they say. I'll be informed in case he makes it—and, of course, in case he doesn't.

"What's your number?" they ask.

Michael has been secured with shoulder, chest, pelvis, and leg straps to the stretcher. And yet, he tries to raise a hand. By instinct, I take it to mean, "Don't give it to them."

I don't want to become overly suspicious of these first responders. After all, they risk their own health to save ours. Even so, all I say is, "I'll call you."

All three of them raise an eyebrow under their Mylar face shields. "As you wish."

The back doors of the ambulance open, casting a gaping shadow that swallows Michael as the paramedics lift him inside. All the while, I hear him moaning. It's the same utterance, over and over again.

If only I knew what he means by that.

More.

*

Lights are still aglow over the kitchen table where we ate last night. I turn them off, and a mood descends heavily upon me, too painful to name. The best I can do is *loneliness*. I refuse to call it *fear* and don't want to admit, even to myself, that I may lose my dearest friend.

Rarely do I tell him what he means to me. Rarely do I use any terms of endearment, which now I come to regret. Even worse, my last words to him rose out of rage. "I'm so angry," I blurted out, a moment before he was hit. "I can't even begin to tell you how angry I am... Don't you *sweetheart* me."

Now, this memory becomes unbearably sharp. It gnaws at me. I hope it doesn't torment him, too.

Does Michael know how much I care about him? Does he trust —despite my flare-up—that he is the one I burn to embrace, the one I love? Was this our last time together? Will there be another moment, another chance for me to open my heart?

Will there be a future for us?

I imagine his voice, tinged with tongue-in-cheek humor. "Not if your Ma has anything to say about it."

I wipe my eyes. Then come doubts of a different kind.

Why did I let these men carry him away? Should I have demanded to stay by his side? Should I have insisted they leave him with me, so he might recover at home? And what if they were not who they presented themselves to be? How were they able to come here so quickly, even before I ended the 911 call? What if they worked hand-in-hand with whoever shot him in the first place?

A shiver goes down my spine.

"Someone must have noticed me poking around," Michael said. "He had me followed. His men destroyed my Tesla—but spared me. For now."

Wracked with guilt for letting them take him out of my sight, I tell myself to just stop it. This agony is merely the result of a sleepless night, filled with trying events.

I call UCLA Medical Center, ask about Michael Morse, but they don't have any information on a patient by that name, not yet. I'll do it again, later.

Next I contact the police again to give them the information they asked for about the shooting. They don't say it, but I get a distinct impression they see it as part of the general unrest. The only promising thing about the conversation is that they recognize my name as it is associated with an open case of identity theft. So I know an investigation has started.

On my way out of Michael's place, I pass once again through the empty garage. Its blue walls, dimly lit by sunrise, press even more sadness into me. And there, in the corner where Michael fell, something glints at me. His cellphone. It must have fallen here by mishap.

Don't accidents have some purpose in the grand scheme of things? I stare at the device. What would Michael bid me do, now that I'm armed with it?

Banged as a result of his collapse, the cellphone has a long hairline crack. It runs diagonally, then zigzags near the bottom of the image through the castors of the pictured ICU bed, formerly occupied by the head of a criminal organization that abducted me.

What would Michael do, faced with his reported death?

Oh, no question about it! He would start poking around to uncover the death certificate, if any, and the location of the corpse. And he would carefully record his findings, so as to share them later with me.

I have no doubt. That is what Michael meant by "There's more."

Now that he's wounded, I can follow through on his search, play out what happened, what his video camera captured. I can do it either on the palm-size display of his cellphone—or in a full-scale simulation that will let me walk through it. Virtually.

First, I need to block the blindingly piercing rays of the rising sun. I lower the garage door to a close. Under its bottom edge, a pencil of light rolls in, emitting a subtle glow. So the space is not as dark as it should ideally be. An impression of its blue walls will remain concretely visible behind the virtual environment.

Oh well, I'll just have to ignore what's real.

By accident, I press a button on his cellphone, which causes the ICU bed to materialize in midair right here in front of me. Oh, this is way too easy! Am I lucky or what?

The time stamp of the video recording—9:27am Pacific Daytime—along with the date float overhead just under the virtual ceiling, under the real one. With this double vision, I feel as if I exist in two instances of time all at once. Past and present.

And something else, something completely new appears out of the blue haze of the garage: a faint crack, traveling diagonally through thin air from the top corner on one side to the bottom corner of the other, ending with a zigzag that cuts through the bed.

And in the middle of that crack appears something that seems utterly weird. A translucent hand.

The thumb has a long, tapered shape, and there is an old scar at the side of the wrist, which is how I know: here is Michael. Correction: here was Michael. Last week.

Instinctively, I reach out to the recorded memory of his hand. But without my VR glove, which I forgot to wear, and the tactile sensors woven into its fabric, my fingers go right through his, missing him entirely. His palm gives no resistance against mine, his skin—no warmth, which dispels the illusion of what I desperately long for. A touch.

Meanwhile, his hand is pushing open the door, and I step out to the virtual corridor. I follow where it points and turn this corner and that until reaching an unfamiliar back exit.

Masked guards in black suits pace to and fro out there. They are guiding a huge vehicle into a parking position. It's a Hino 26' Reefer with gigantic ribbed tires, aluminum roof, and an ad plastered onto its side. It reads,

> *Transporting perishables demands reliable refrigerated transportation. We're well aware of this fact and can deliver the perfect truck for your needs*

For a moment, I wonder what exactly is meant by *perishables*. Ice Cream? Vegetables? Poultry?

The answer soon becomes clear. Around me, masked medical workers wheel out one body after another, each covered in a zipped white plastic bag, on one gurney after another. A forklift operator carefully raises each pallet in turn onto the corrugated metal floor of the truck.

This, to me, is a harrowing sight.

I've heard, of course, that hospitals in several pandemic epicenters passed a tipping point in the fight against the virus. The relentless climb in infections forced them to store corpses in makeshift morgues such as trucks, refrigerated to delay decomposition.

Seeing this play out before my eyes is quite different from knowing it in the abstract. This, I realize, is a war zone. In every city, every town, every village, the number of casualties is mounting, with no end in sight.

While these thoughts flood my mind, a subtle zipping sound startles me into confusion. What is this? What's happening to the scene? Why has it become obscured? Where the hell am I now?

Then, it dawns on me. I understand what Michael must have done to achieve this frightening effect, virtual as it may be, of near-blindness. He must have found an empty body bag, stepped into the thing and pulled the zipper upon himself, perhaps to escape being noticed. His view, as recorded by his camera, became shrouded.

The masked guards, the fork lift operator, the medical workers in full body gear, the piles of the deceased, the empty gurneys, even the huge truck, are all veiled away. Their sounds are now dim, muffled into near-silence.

But somehow I sense being lifted, then lowered into the truck. The one thing I'm thankful for is not being able to feel its hard, corrugated floor under me.

My teeth begin to chatter.

The only way for me to avoid panic is by letting myself be carried away—except that by drifting into this blankness, my mind is overwhelmed by more and more elements of distress. Immersed in virtual nothingness, the notion of body bags at my sides makes me recoil. But such is the power of bringing to life, with digital preciseness, just what Michael saw, what he sensed. In my mind, I become him. We become one.

The prospect of being buried alive makes my heart palpitate with intolerable horror. I feel the oppression of the lungs, the flaring of the nostrils. I try to draw in oxygen, even by the most minute whiff—only to be stifled by the thought of fumes from the other bodies.

Even worse, I'm overcome by the inescapable thought of worms eating at the flesh, swarming inside the body bags to my left and right. I am thirsty for air, air flowing freely just outside this garment of death.

Michael must have been inflicted with the same anxiety that overtakes me now. Who would come to save me? Who could even guess my fate?

Meanwhile I sense, by its muffled ramble, the engine revving up.

The one bright spot I cling to is a new appreciation for Michael. Who knows how often these body bags are disinfected. Hiding inside one of them may pose danger. In spite of this risk, he took it upon himself to follow the Russian and record the descent to his final resting place. All for my sake, for my peace-of-mind.

If Michael could do it, so can I!

As the back door of the truck slams shut, the translucent impression of his hand reappears. To my relief, it begins to pull down the zipper. Then it freezes, as the view is unveiled. In a blink, the body bag opposite me starts to stir.

I rub my eyes in wonder.

What is this? The rising of the dead? For a moment I expect to see sinews being laid upon dry bones, and flesh miraculously forming upon them, soon to be covered with skin.

But no. What is playing out before me is no miracle. Rather, it is a correction of a former error in judgement. Someone who I —and everyone else—mistook for a stiff, wiggles free out of the bag.

Chapter 6

Rising to his feet in the unlit interior of the refrigerated truck is a barefoot figure, quite imposing even from a distance. He has the build of a bear and a few shaggy skin patches across his shoulder blades to complement it.

This is when I become so immersed, so swept into the virtual reality scene playing out against the blue walls of the empty garage, that I forget it depicts events dating back to last week. I forget it was recorded by Michael, at great risk to his life. I see it from his point of view, which has become mine. I am him. Virtually.

The simulation, conjured by a click on his cellphone, is all too convincing. Lying on a floor of a virtual truck, I spy on the figure through a tiny hole in my body bag. A digital timestamp shows a past date floating over my head. This, for me, is now.

Meanwhile, the burly man leans against the insulated panel of the truck, perhaps to regain his balance. His toe tag scrapes against the corrugated metal floor. It flaps for a second right in front of my eyes—but not long enough for me to read it.

Despite a careful look around the space, he seems unaware of being recorded. Shrugging off the hospital sheets in which he's been wrapped, he stuffs them back into his plastic body bag so it appears full.

Then, the man cups his ear as if listening to some sound beyond the annoying swish of body bags, lined along the length of the truck. With a slight rustle, they're shaking side to side to the rhythm of the drive. But other than the indeterminate hum of the engine, nothing else stands out.

The only noise that starts torturing my imagination is the constant hiss of dead silence. It is against that backdrop that I sense the tumultuous pounding of my heart and the beat of blood pulsing in my ears.

Can the man hear these sounds, too? Will he turn around to me? Will he take note of my eye—or rather, the eye of the video camera—peeking out of my body bag? Will he rush over and crush it? Oh, I can just imagine him plonking his heel on it, and —*clonk!*

Will he zip my bag to a hermetic close, depriving me of air? Cringing in fear, I can't help but hold my breath.

Now, that can't last forever. Against my better judgement, I end up gasping. If I'm lucky, the shriek of air rushing to my lungs will be engulfed by the rumble of the truck as it is turning a corner. I feel it in my bones, the spin of the rubbery tires, the hum of the motor, the beat of the road, and above all—the charge ahead at full speed toward some destination, who knows where.

In my anxiety, I feel an overwhelming temptation to lapse into an insensible state. Oh, how I long for sweet rest! Eternal sleep may be waiting for me beyond the moment of drawing a last breath. The thought of it, alluring as it may be, is somewhat strange. Yet it comes to soothe me, as if it were a violin string vibrating softly in a misty blue haze.

On second thought, no. I refuse to succumb to it.

Meanwhile, the man has opened a container. Apparently, it holds loose personal effects which, according to procedure, are stored separately from the remains.

From there, he grabs a plaid shirt, flings it over his shoulders, left sleeve, right. Then, pants. Then, to my utter surprise, he pulls out the most incredible costume, one that will allow him to become inconspicuous once the truck arrives at the unloading site.

What the man is stepping into is a translucent plastic full body suit, complete with a Mylar face shield, mouth and nose covering, and gloves, the kind medical workers would wear when treating highly contagious patients. His plan is clever. I get it. Upon arrival, he'll simply pretend to sort out the body bags like other medical workers. Sooner or later, he'll find an opportunity to slip away, unrecognized and unnoticed.

Despite a growing suspicion, I can't determine with certainty who he is, but tell myself to be patient. Well, what other choice do I have?

After all, this I know: Medical examiners can get fired if they release the wrong decedent. To prevent this, they place not only a toe tag or an ankle band on the corpse, but also a tag on its body bag. The names on these tags must match each other when the body is conveyed to the funeral home. So, once this man extricates himself from here—clearly, that's what he intends to do—I can examine the tag left behind on his body bag.

Well, no. Too late for that. The man has just loosened his tags —from both his body bag and his big toe—and is scratching his head, perhaps figuring out how to use them to his advantage, how to cause the most mischief. His footfalls are coming closer.

Thud, thud, thud, he swaggers across the floor, stepping over this body bag and that, until—oh no!—stumbling over mine. He lands on top of me, hard. I clump my jaws together so as not to utter a cry. Then, regaining my presence of mind, I give myself a pat on the shoulder.

Mentally.

He spits something out loud. Sounds like a juicy Russian curse.

I don't even comprehend the language, but what else can it be but *shit*?

Just the word I was looking for.

The man rolls over to the floor, dusts off his knees, and unzips the body bag lying just next to mine. Inside is a wrinkled human carcass with black toes. Speaking about toes, I'm so glad—did I say this already?—that the software that supports this virtual simulation has not been upgraded to a version that includes smell.

Bending over the carcass, the Russian replaces both of its tags —the one on its toe as well as the one on its bag—with his.

Then, he straightens and stretches over to the air conditioning control panel mounted on the insulated panel. To my astonishment, he turns it off. This guy doesn't like frigid temperatures. And why should he? He's not in Russia anymore.

In Los Angeles county, the season makes a big difference in the speed of putrefaction. During the summer, a corpse starts bloating within two days. It is facially identifiable for only one. So when the wrinkled carcass is prepared for burial, the only evidence of its identity will be these tags. The wrong ones, now dangling from its body bag in plain view.

I know the name printed on them all too well.

Vlad Komarov. Age 37.

The man formerly known as Vlad heads for the double-wing rear doors of the truck. With a grunt, he presses his weight against them. Shouldn't there be a latch on the outside, to secure the contents of the truck?

Did someone neglect to lock the truck properly? No. That's unlikely. Did Vlad have an accomplice? Maybe one of his gang members infiltrated the hospital pretending to be a medic or a nurse, printed the toe tag, forged the death certificate, loaded him on the truck, and loosened the door latch so Vlad could slip out. I know this is speculation, and quite wild at that—but how else could this getaway succeed? Who knows, his accomplice may have even provided him with a weapon.

The doors begin to sway open. Through the gap between them, I catch sight of the road rattling away. Buildings swing around street corners before shrinking into the distance.

Then—when I least expect it—a ring.

It shakes me out of my deep immersion in the scene, but not before the man turns his head over his shoulder and casts a sharp look, scanning the darkened space.

For a second I think he's heard the ring, too—only to remind myself that he can't. This scene is merely a record of past actions. I alone can hear the sounds of the present. I alone am real.

Even so, something must have drawn his attention at the time of the recording. I see him turning back swiftly, aiming a Russian M1895 Nagant revolver directly at me.

No, not at me—at Michael.

Gripped by horror, the cellphone drops out of my hand.

In a blink, the entire virtual scene disintegrates. The interior of the refrigerated truck, its air conditioning control panel, its half-open double-wing rear doors, the corrugated floor, lined with body bags, and Vlad stepping on them, revolver in hand, all turn into scattering pixels, into dust.

But the ringing goes on, on and on, incessantly.

Utterly confused, rubbing my eyes as if coming out of a dream, I look around me at the blue walls of the garage. This nausea I feel, this cyber sickness, is caused by plunging into virtual reality. Based on previous experiences, my daze can last for several hours after getting out of the simulation. I take a deep breath and try to relax.

But then, the ringing. Won't it stop? Won't someone pick it up already? Who's cellphone is this?

Oh, mine.

It's Rita, calling me on FaceTime. "You all right?" she asks.

"Of course," I say, shakily. "Why?"

"Because, I want to show you something. Tell me what you think of it."

She texts me a grainy black-and-white video, probably taken from a surveillance camera, showing a woman who seems to be in her early twenties. She is opening her duffle bag at the teller station of a bank. Her hair is cropped short with spiky layers at the top, just my style. The shadow of her long lashes flutters over the eyes, but can't blot out the sparkle in them. Looking at her is like looking at myself in a mirror.

The last time I visited a branch of Wells Fargo was over a year ago, when I opened my savings account. Was this when this video was taken?

"Well?" says Rita.

"Well what?" I say, with a shrug. "I looked smashing back then, if I say so myself."

She shakes her head. "So, you think it's you?"

"I do."

Her plucked eyebrow shoots up to her hairline. "Think again."

Chapter 7

A bit disoriented, I rub my eyes. It doesn't help my cybersickness dissipate any faster. "Well, what d'you mean, *think again?*"

Rita shakes her head with great vigor, to the point that it nearly rolls off the cellphone screen. "Oh dear." She puffs her cheeks. "Do I have to spell it out? It took great pain to get that surveillance video. Concentrate, dear. Watch it more carefully. Just look at her—"

"You mean, me? Look at me?"

"No. She isn't you."

"You're kidding, right?"

Rita folds her arms, her face stern as if to match her stubbornness to mine. "Whatever gave you that idea?"

By now, I'm out of the garage and into my Escape, hoping to regain my focus once I start driving. I know, I know. Bad idea. But things must get moving along, even if you happen to put them out of order.

I need to check if Michael is in UCI Medical Center. Need to bring him home. Need to see my mother. And Pa. Need to bring them some groceries, so they don't risk spending time with other shoppers. Need to go back to LA and resume my job search.

Leaping in, Browny places his paws on my knees and gives me a sullen look, as if knowing how confused I feel, as if begging me to come to my senses. He licks my nose and, for extra emphasis, goes as far as slobbering all over me.

I've slipped my cellphone into its holder and propped it against the dashboard. With a single click, I alternate between watching Rita, who has just facepalmed—twice—to show her frustration with me, and watching the woman in the grainy, black-and-white surveillance video.

At first glance, that woman's face looks like a reflection of mine, and her hair has the exact same wisps curling around the slender neck. I can almost feel them tickling my own skin.

Glancing at the overhead mirror, I marvel at the spot-on similarity between me and her, except that right now, my hair is messier and my eyes—droopier, with black circles under them, remnants of a sleepless night.

I flip back to see Rita. A bit red in the face, she seems annoyed with me. Testy. We know each other well, so I can say without a doubt that both of us need the first jolt of caffeine to face our daily grind.

"I beg you," she says. "For your own good, take one more look—"

"Can't you see?" Exasperated, I raise my hands in the air. "This is me, for sure. A few months ago, I think."

"This video was shot last week."

"Now, *that* I doubt—"

"Oh dear. Wake up already, will you?" Rita sets her fists on her waist, elbows pointing out. "What's the matter with you this morning?"

"Nothing—"

"D'you smoke?"

"Of course not."

"Did you ever?"

"No!"

"But *that woman* does."

I study *that woman* again, this time carefully. There's no cigarette butt between her fingers, and the only thing dangling from her lips is a lovely smile. "Really? How can you tell?"

"Ash, I talked to the bank teller."

"And?"

"And he couldn't forget the smell of her smoke-impregnated clothes. It wafted over the partition between them."

Rolling my eyes, I hold on to a mindset of defending myself. How dare Rita accuse me of a sin—even if it's only smoking? I may have many vices, but that's not one of them.

She seems as if she's itching to nudge me. "Well?"

"Well, the teller is wrong." The only time I tried smoking was when I took a drag of a cigarette from some boy, whose name I can't even recall, back in high school. "That smell must have come from someone else."

Rita drags a hand down her face. "Oh, Ash." She sighs. "That woman may have copied your haircut, may have glued some false eyelashes and painted her face to resemble you. She walked across the floor with the same sexy bounce to her step—but for all her efforts, she couldn't hide her habit."

"What habit?"

"See that smile? Her teeth were stained nicotine yellow, the telltale sign of a regular smoker."

"Oh really?" The incredulity in my tone must be driving Rita nuts. "And you can tell that from a black-and-white image?"

Rita frowns.

For a minute I sense she's about to stab the disconnect button. Instead, she draws a startled breath, but before she has the chance to gather a few words into a sentence, I flip over to the video and catch sight of something that—to my dismay—proves me wrong.

And boy, how I hate being wrong!

The woman in the video must have loosened the drawstring of her duffle bag. Its opening comes to light, revealing a small pack of cigarettes, tucked inside. Camel.

"Oh, Rita, I'm so sorry," I cry. "You're right!"

For a while, Rita is quiet. I suppose she's fighting an urge to say, "Told you so." When at last she says it, a victorious smile licks at the corners of her mouth.

I freeze the video, zoom into the paused image, and suddenly recognize one facial feature that does not belong to me.

The cheeks, sunken.

In a snap, I realize who I'm dealing with: the woman from Point Dume, the one I fished out of the water a couple of weeks ago. I recall Michael carrying her in his arms along the beach, her knee over his left elbow, her foot dangling in the air, blood oozing. I remember her head lolling over his right shoulder and, with every one of his steps, shadows sliding in and out of her hollow cheeks.

But in this video, just look at her! She's undergone some miraculous changes. Her scalp used to be bald but has somehow sprouted hair, and her figure used to be flat-chested but has turned curvaceous. When she washed ashore, I thought at first that it was a man. No longer can I make that mistake.

Of course, there are plenty of other mistakes to be made. Leave it to me to stumble into another one of them.

"Hello, *Ms. Voola*," I mutter, calling her by the one word she muttered in response to every one of my questions.

Rita leans in. "Is that her name? Really?"

I shrug. "No. Wish I knew it."

For a while, we say nothing.

I turn the key to start the engine, preparing to let go as soon as the engine has started. Instead, it starts stuttering. Sigh. This ignition problem creeps up more often than not. I hope it takes care of itself, somehow, because how can I afford fixing it?

Browny rests his head on the passenger seat and claps his paws over his eyes. He must sense how worried I am.

At last, Rita says, "She stole your hairstyle and copied the shape of your eyebrows, not to mention your breasts."

My breath catches in my thudding chest. "What she snatched away is something far more important. My identity."

"So sorry," says Rita, her voice softening.

"That makes two of us."

"It takes some study, and some practice on top of that, to walk and talk just the way you do. She must be an actress. Quite good at what she does."

"No wonder she fooled even me."

"Even worse," says Rita. "She fooled the bank teller, too."

I flip back to watch the last segment of the video. There, *Ms. Voola* presents a driver's license—mine—then accepts a stack of hundred dollar bills in a currency strap, which she stuffs deep into her duffle bag.

"That's your money she's walking out with," says Rita. "See the way she's winking, over her shoulder? That's her way of telling you to kiss it goodbye."

A groan wells in my throat. "Oh no! That's my entire savings. I'm going to get it out of her if it kills me."

"You be careful, Ash—"

I snort a laugh. "She's the one who should be careful, because I'm coming after her."

Rita waves her hand in dismissal. "Ah, you don't even know her name."

"I'll figure it out," I promise. "I'll find her, just you watch me! And when I do, I'm going to punch her lights out."

Chapter 8

My grip on the steering wheel is strong, perhaps too strong—by contrast to my grip on the rolling disaster called my life. I tell myself to just hold on, just be me, but that has never been trickier, now that someone else is a contender not only for my name but also for who I am.

As I drive to Ma's home, my knuckles turn bone-white no matter how often I try to relax them. Of course, *Ms. Voola* is to blame. I feel an undeniable urge to wring her neck for stealing my money along with my identity. Who knows what other surprises that woman has in store for me.

Unfortunately, it's one thing to promise I'll get my hands on her— quite another to actually do it, especially when all I know about that woman with any degree of certainty is that she has sunken cheeks. That's the only facial feature she failed to disguise while playing the role of Ashley Winters at the bank.

Clearly, *Ms. Voola* has a penchant for acting. She's good enough to be a professional, given her performance mimicking the way I walk and talk, not to mention the makeup and hairdo job that fooled even my own eyes.

I turn a corner and nosedive into sudden despair. What I'm looking for is an actress with sunken cheeks, probably residing in LA. That's like looking for a needle in a haystack of needles. A prickly proposition. Chances are I'll come out of it empty-handed.

I marvel at the skill of that woman and fear her in the breath of whispering, "Who are you, *Ms. Voola?*"

How long has she been studying me? In other words, was it simply by accident that I stumbled upon her during a casual walk on the beach, or did she plan it well ahead of time? Over and over again, I picture her hand reaching into my purse to snatch my driver's license and health insurance card. Did she pretend to have lost consciousness, knowing I would let her get close to me—close enough to steal what's mine?

On my way to Irvine, I call the hospital. All they tell me is that they're overwhelmed right now, there's no news about how Michael Morse is doing, and call later. Even though that's not much, I utter a sigh of relief. At least, now I know he's been checked in.

Up until now I've been tormented by the suspicion that he might have been taken away by some gang members pretending to be paramedics. These days, it's hard to know for sure who's who, all because of the masks. No wonder my imagination goes into overdrive.

I make a quick stop to buy some groceries for my mother, then head for her place. Having parked the Escape, I let Browny out. He leaps out and races me to her door.

Wiping my feet on the doormat, I feel like a child again. And I know why I'm here. What I need is a hug.

*

"Ashley!" Ma says, placing a palm over her heart as if to stop a wild pounding. "What are you doing here?"

I shrug. "Just dropping by."

She fills a dish with some water and sets it on the floor for Browny. While he's lapping it, her eyes bore into mine. "Dear, is something wrong?"

"No, Ma, I just missed you," I say, stunned for a second by the sight of her face. It's covered in a green layer. Strangely enough, it reminds me of the good times in our family. Pa would come home to find my mother wearing an avocado facial with slices of cucumbers over her eyes and a towel wrapped around her hair.

I remember. He would raise his hands as if to praise the Lord for this wonderful gift, the gift of being married to beauty in the flesh. Goes to show you that when it comes to the opposite sex, men are not all that smart. Which he proved, years later, by divorcing my mother and marrying a younger version of her.

I bring in the groceries I've bought on my way here to save her the trouble of going to the stores. Ma rolls up her sleeves and embarks on her routine, which she developed long before the start of the pandemic. First, she wipes the bags clean while holding them in the air at arms-length. Then, she fishes out each one of the products and wipes it top to bottom, as if it were a naughty baby about to soil her counter.

Afterwards, Ma runs to the kitchen faucet and rinses her face clean. The facial hasn't worked the magic she must have been hoping for. It hasn't smoothed out the years. I'm the last person to tell her that. My heart aches for her. She looks more fragile than ever. More crinkled, too. The marionette lines at either side of her mouth have deepened since the last time I saw her.

Having wiped her face dry with the dishtowel, her hand goes to her teased hair, hastily fixing it. "Why didn't you tell me you're coming?"

"Sorry, Ma. I decided to come on the spur of a moment—"

"Something is the matter, Ashley. Don't you try to deny it."

"Can't I come here, just because?"

She crosses her arms. "Because what, exactly?"

"Because." The thought of food stabs at my gut. All of a sudden, I realize how hungry I am. "I love your Challah bread."

She wraps her arms around me and gives me a squeeze. And for the first time in days, I'm happy.

"Ah," she says, this time beaming with pride. "It's my secret recipe."

We take opposite seats at the kitchen table. "Yes, Ma. I know."

"Want to learn how to make it?"

"I do."

Ma fishes a crumb from a fold in the tablecloth and rubs it down to nothing between her wrinkled fingers. Then, she places her hand over mine and gives me a gentle pat. It feels so good.

"The most important ingredient," she says, "is time. The dough must rise not once, not twice, but three times—"

"Oh. Time. That's something I don't really have right now, Ma." The moment these words leave my lips, I wish I could take them back.

The grin falls away from her lips. "I knew it." And in a blink, she starts sobbing. Loudly.

Taken by surprise, I say. "Please, Ma, don't take it so hard."

She sniffs between one wail and another, but not long enough to answer.

"Oh, stop crying," I plead. "So sorry. The last thing I want to do is hurt your feelings."

She presses the dishtowel to her face, and her shoulders shake with each little moan.

I can't help but ask, "Is it just because of the Challah?"

"No, Ashley," she whimpers. "Not just that."

"What, then?"

She waves her hand as if to say, oh, it's nothing, dear, don't mind me, but then come the words, "Oh, what can I say? It's everything. Too much is happening, all at once."

"Like what, Ma?"

"Well, have you seen the boarded-up shop windows? And the riot police in the streets? And then, there's that which you can't see, but I know it's lurking out there. I picture it creeping closer and closer to my doorstep. The virus. It drives me indoors, where I feel so isolated, so alone. I'm not good at being a recluse."

"That's why I'm here, to keep you company—"

"What can I do?" She wipes her nose, sniffles. "Vacuum? Dust the furniture? Clean the shower with a fine toothbrush?"

"Please, Ma. Just try to relax."

"How can I?" She whimpers. "Oh, I'm too old for PMS, but feel like I've had it for days. A massive anxiety over the sad state of everything. Even chocolate cannot fix this crap."

She goes on complaining that the country is not the same as it used to be. Neither is the world. Neither is she, for that matter, but I'm not going to be the one to tell her that.

After a while, Ma recovers into a little smile, while still dabbing the wet corners of her eyes. "I don't know what came over me. I suppose it's because of the suicide, next door."

"What?"

"Oh, you don't know? My neighbor. You may remember him. A short, hunched man with narrow shoulders. He used to work as a dermatologist, Dr. Leo Cohen—"

"Vaguely. He had a curly mustache, right?"

"What a shame," she says, over my words. "He blew his brains out."

"Oh no! Why?"

"His identity got stolen and his bank account—emptied."

My jaw drops, and Ma presses on. "If you ask me, Dr. Cohen died not of the bullet—but of the embarrassment."

Mouth agape, I'm still speechless.

My mother shakes her head in utter dismay. "All the windows in the building rattled at the sound of that shot. I ran to his door. Strangely enough it wasn't locked, so I nudged it open and found Dr. Cohen there, in his study—oh, those glassy eyes! I'll never forget that look, never, as long as I live! And then," she says, with a shudder, "when I bent over him, he was still warm to the touch."

"Did he leave a note?"

"I couldn't find one, and when the police came, neither could they."

"Then, how can you be so sure that was the reason he took his own life?"

"Because."

"Because what?"

"Because, he told me yesterday—just as I waved hello to him from my kitchen window—that someone got his retirement savings out of Pacific Premier Bank. Who, I ask you, would do such a thing? My God, what is the world coming to?"

Ma unfolds *The Orange County Register*, slaps it on the table, and shoves it over to me. "See? Read this."

I scan the page. First article, *Long Beach Police Make Arrests in Party Shooting that Killed 3*. Next one, *Riverside Man Arrested on Suspicion of Kill-and-Run*. And the third, underlined in red ink, *Irvine Police calls for the public's help to identify a suspect in a criminal activity at Pacific Premier Bank*.

This last article includes a photo of said suspect. He seems to be a in his mid-fifties, wearing a curly mustache, just like the one I remember on Dr. Cohen. The impostor is dressed in a starched, long-sleeve white shirt with a crisp collar and a red tie, and carrying a spiffy leather attaché briefcase. His shoulders are narrow and head— bald. Even as he gives a sly smile and nods to the bank teller, his cheeks remain hollow.

I bite my lip so as not to cry.

"Don't bite your lip," says Ma. "It's a nasty habit. Maybe you're hungry?"

She leans into her feet with a heavy sigh, then brings me a glass of cool lemonade with ice cubes dancing inside and dewdrops beading all around. I drain it. Without wasting a moment, she refills the glass and sets a plate before me. It's heaped with her homemade chocolate chip cookies, hot from the oven.

Golden brown around the edges, the cookie melts in my mouth. I stuff my face with more crumbling sweet nothings, intent on holding back any disturbing thoughts. Even so, they keep hissing in the back of my mind.

So, *Ms Voola*, is that you, this time here in Irvine, performing the same old tricks? Boy, you've been working overtime lately, running up and down the state of California whenever money can be grabbed from fools, innocent fools like me and like Dr. Cohen, who have only themselves to blame for letting their guard down.

✳

While Ma is busy packing the rest of the cookies for me in a tin can, and Browny is licking the dog bowl clean, I text Rita a snapshot of the article about the suspect seen at Pacific Premier Bank. Then I step outside and call her.

"Guess what," I say. "The woman who emptied my bank account has just struck again."

"Is that her? I'm not so sure."

"I am."

"Maybe," she says. "Same cheeks. Same sly smile."

"And," I say, "same crime."

"Oh, I don't know. My police friend claims they ran the surveillance image of that woman through facial recognition, but came up empty."

"Strange."

"On a different note, Ash, remember the syringe you picked on the beach?"

"How can I forget?"

"The DNA results are in."

"And?"

"And," says Rita, "I don't want to upset you."

Anxiety starts roiling in my stomach, but no one needs to know that. "Just tell me what you know."

"Are you sitting down?"

"I am."

"They found trace amounts of DNA on the tip of the needle."

"And?"

"And," she says, "it's identical to the DNA found inside you after you were raped."

I gasp.

I wipe my palms on my jeans, I try to say something, anything—but find it impossible.

A moment later, Rita says, "You alright?"

I try to answer, but my trembling lips won't obey me. My mind doesn't, either. Finally I mutter, "Yes. No. I don't know."

How strange. I have no name, not even a face for the thug who raped me. I wouldn't recognize him if he passed me on the street. All I remember is the white of his eye, marbled with tortuous veins, and his voice, heavy with a Russian accent.

What blows my mind is the coincidence—his DNA on the syringe, coupled with the fact that *Ms. Voola* stepped on it—which suggests that both of them were at Pointe Dume at roughly the same time. Do they know each other? Are they partners in crime? Or else, is she his newest victim?

I end the call, then go kiss my mother goodbye and promise to spend more time with her next time, so I can learn her baking secrets. She hands me a shopping bag filled with envelopes, large and small.

"What's that?" I ask.

"Don't you remember? When you left Irvine, you filled out a postal address change to forward your mail to me. I removed all the junk mail. These," she says, shaking the bag so its contents give a rustle, "are what's left."

Armed with the bag and with her tin can, I open the door and head to my Escape. Light drizzle hangs in the air, which is unusual for the sunny summers of California and perfect for anyone in gloom.

The heels of Ma's sensible shoes clink and clunk behind as she scrambles to catch up with Browny and me. "Wait! It's raining!"

"Oh, Ma, it's just a drizzle."

"Ashley, I don't want you to catch a cold."

She holds her flowery umbrella over me so I wouldn't melt and tucks me, ever so carefully, into the driver's seat. Her mission accomplished, my mother scuttles back. In a minute, she'll be leaning out of her kitchen window to wave goodbye.

I turn the key and glide smoothly away, but my mind remains stuck in a rut. There is some sinister connection between the thug and *Ms. Voola*. If only I knew what it was.

Chapter 9

I'd like to believe that I don't scare easily, but when a red 2020 Chevrolet Impala appears in the rearview mirror time and again, following me closely through several stop signs and traffic lights, my heart skips a beat. I step on the gas. The road is slippery because of the morning rain, which may explain why the Chevrolet sails forward all of a sudden and bumps my rear fender.

"Knock, knock," I mutter, trying to make light of it. "Who's there?"

The only answer I get is a second attempt to ram me.

Gritting my teeth, I clamp the steering wheel and go for evasive maneuvers. Having watched car chases in the movies, I've had plenty of couch practice. Still, given my clunky Escape, shaking off an aggressive driver is a challenge, which forces me to pull out all the stops. I swerve frantically between lanes, around intersections, in and out of side streets I don't even know.

Not that I'm afraid of whoever it might be, trailing me with such dogged determination. But I don't like being watched and —for some time now—I have a persistent sense that I am. I recall what Michael told me when his car exploded in flames. "What happened to my Tesla is merely a warning. There's more to come."

In a flash, the Chevrolet overtakes me. For a second, its red shine blinds my eyes. Squinting, I think I spot the driver's profile. The cheek is sunken.

The side of her vehicle grates—as if by accident—against mine. Then, the Chevrolet slips back and follows me from a distance of three cars. The murky silhouette of the driver is now barely readable behind her darkened windshield. Is she biding her time before pouncing on me at full force?

I heave a sigh, guessing she's not going to wait forever.

If I'm not scared, perhaps I should be.

To my surprise, the red Chevrolet recedes into the traffic behind me. At first, its chrome license plate frame, decorated with the classic bowtie logo, still peeks out in the background behind this or that car. I see it in my rearview mirror—but not long enough to decipher the reflection of its number. I promise myself to practice reading things in reverse, if I'm lucky enough to get out of this tight spot.

After a while, a fleeting red blur can be spotted in the distance, but only if I screw up my eyes. By the time I take the onramp, the Chevrolet is nowhere to be seen.

California State Route 133 connects Irvine through the San Joaquin Hills to Laguna Beach, which is where Pa lives nowadays, divorced from my mother and separated from his current wife. I miss him. I long for the safe feeling that wraps over me in his company. And I wonder if—in these troubled times—he enjoys his newfound solitude, or else, if he suffers the isolation that comes with being alone.

∗

Pa's one-bedroom rental sits on a hill. From a distance, it looks like a quaint garden shed. I park my Escape by the curb, gather the grocery bags I packed full of food for him and, with Browny bounding behind me, climb the uneven stone walkway leading up to his front deck.

Slumped on a dilapidated wooden bench, my father seems to have nodded off. His eyes are shut to the view of a rainbow that starts clarifying over the ocean. Only when my shadow falls across the newspaper folded in his lap, and the sound of my footfalls comes to a halt, he stirs.

Running a hand through his silver hair, "Good to see you, Ash," Pa says, without the least bit of surprise. "I had a feeling you'd come."

"Funny, I had the same feeling."

Then, I tell him that I've just self-quarantined for a couple of weeks. "Me too," he says. "I've seen no one for what seems like ages."

I tell him Ma sends her regards and hopes to see him. He says Heather, his current wife who lives in Clearwater, Florida, asks about me, on the rare occasions she answers his calls.

Then, he stretches into a yawn. Every morning, the *Orange County Register* is delivered to his doorstep. Without fail, reading it puts him to sleep. Today is no exception.

He points at the headline. "Read it out loud for me, Ash, will you?"

"But Pa, your reading glasses are right here, on your head—"

"Never mind my reading glasses. They're no good, anyway."

So, I pick up the newspaper and spread it out. "You like mafia stories, right?"

"Sure do!"

"Here's one. Gangsters belonging to Armenian Power, a highly organized international crime group, were found to be involved in the 2010 Medicaid fraud case and the 2011 FBI-led Operation Power Outage."

He shakes his head. "What is the world coming to?"

I feel like kissing his wrinkled brow but hold myself back, then glance at the next sentence. "Their illegal activities ranged from bank fraud to identity theft."

I put the newspaper aside and squat to rub my Golden Retriever between the ears. The last thing I want to discuss with my dad is that my own bank account has been compromised, my own identity stolen.

Instead, I go for the mundane. "I got you some chocolate chip cookies. Also, bags of rice and lentils. Peaches and plums, too. And a few cartons of almond milk."

"What about cereal?"

"Frosted Flakes and Honey Nut Cheerios."

Pa smiles, and we carry the bags to his kitchenette, where I help him unpack the groceries. The shelves are sparsely stocked. I'm happy he has some food now, or he'll start skipping meals.

The kitchenette is open to the living room, which doubles as a bedroom. I sweep my eyes across the gloomy space. The sofa is covered in a rumpled sheet of some indeterminate color, with a punched-in pillow propped up at one end. The other end is draped by a flannel blanket, most of which has slipped to the floor. On top of a narrow dresser, pill bottles are neatly arranged next to a box of moist eyelid wipes, between a glucose meter and a blood pressure monitor.

There's a clunky end table next to the sofa. There, on a stack of books, an old-fashioned watch with a worn-out leather strap is silently ticking away the seconds. A small wastebasket stands in the corner, filled with drafts: crumpled sheets of failed poetry. The entire scene is a study in loneliness.

I open a window to air out the place, then both of us return to the front deck. Here, Browny is sprawled under the bench, his paws covering his eyes, about to doze off.

We lean over the wooden railing of the deck. Raindrops drip, with a brilliant sparkle, off the leaves of Hopi Crape Myrtle shrubs. Their branches, in full bloom, frame a hazy view of the Pacific Ocean. Out there, waves roll ashore one after another, crested with glinting foam.

"Pa," I say, "how are you these days?"

And he says, "Busy."

"Doing what?"

"Writing my memoirs."

"Pa, you've been saying this for the past ten years."

"Have I? Then, it must be true."

I hesitate to ask, "What's taking so long?"

"Spilling words on paper is easy." Pa chuckles. "The hard part is to spill them in the right order."

No doubt, he expects me to ask for a sample of his recent writing, but I can't bring myself to do it. The little I read a few months ago left me with an uneasy feeling. It makes me wince even now.

Using vivid detail, Pa described various scenes in his life, including intimate moments spent behind closed doors not only with my mother but also with other women, which was more than I ever wanted to know. Literary enlightenment is a good thing, in general—but not if I must gain it by being a fly on his bedroom wall.

I remember handing his stack of pages, densely scribbled, back to him without a single word of encouragement, let alone praise. One day, I'm going to regret it. For now, I'm not ready for a full disclosure of his life. He's my father, for crying out loud!

"Don't worry," he says, giving me a knowing look. A sad one. "I'm not going to ask you to read my manuscript."

"I will, Pa. Once you publish it."

By his groan, he's hurt. My father can hear what I left unsaid. He can read my reluctance to get involved in his creative endeavor. I imagine him, pen in hand, forehead furrowing, jotting down his sentences lovingly, meticulously, in his beautiful, slanted longhand. His story will live on through the letters he inks on one page after another—or so he hopes. If only his memories can spring from the paper into a new mind. If only he can find someone to read them.

My heart aches for him. But before I have a chance to take back my refusal, he raises a hand to stop me.

"Forget it," he says. "I found someone who, unlike those closest to me, is more than happy to offer constructive criticism."

"Really, Pa? Who?"

"I met her at a play."

"Which one?"

"*A Midsummer's Night Dream.*"

"Where?"

"At Laguna Playhouse."

This is known for its captivating comedies, dramas, musicals, and standup comedy. Steps away from the Pacific Ocean, it is not too far from here. "But Pa, wasn't it forced to close its doors?"

"It was, when the pandemic started."

"Too bad."

"No more shows for me," he says. "And no more performances for Linda."

"Linda?"

"That's her name."

A new girlfriend, I figure. This time, one with a refined cultural taste. Out loud I just mutter, "Oh."

"It's not what you think."

"It isn't?"

"No, Ash. Granted, I had my share of love affairs. This is not one of them. It's anything but."

I raise an eyebrow.

"Linda is a breast cancer survivor," he says, his tone unusually somber. "Believe me, I'm not interested in her boobs—I mean, she hasn't got any—but her mind is something I admire."

"Since when are you interested in brainy women? I never thought you would be."

"That makes two of us."

"I'm impressed, Pa."

He shrugs. "Linda gives me great editing suggestions. I find them inspiring."

"And no boobs?"

"No. She underwent double mastectomy, a year ago."

"Oh. Sorry to hear it."

We watch the waves in silence for a long time.

Meanwhile, the mention of surgical procedures reminds me to call UCI Medical Center. As I pull out my cellphone, Pa asks, as if he can read my mind, "How's Michael?"

"Not well," I say.

"I like him," says Pa, warmly. "Always did."

I wish Ma would feel the same way. During my visit, she asked me nothing about my boyfriend, a clear indication of just how much she likes him.

If Michael ever asks for my hand—which I think he was about to do when that bullet hit him—we should elope at once, without even mentioning it to her. We should move overseas to some remote location way out of her reach, so my mother won't hound me the rest of my life for not having the wedding she thought I should have, using the caterer and flower shop of her choosing, with a man she would approve. Alas, such a man has not yet been born.

I place a call to the hospital, my third one since Michael was admitted early this morning. My voice cracks when I ask about him. "What's his condition?"

"Please hold," says the receptionist.

Pa cocks his head closer to mine, and we wait together for an answer. For a tense moment that seems like forever, only silence greets both of us.

At last, her voice comes back. "You still there?"

"I am."

"Michael Morse is now in surgery."

"When would he be out?"

"In a couple of hours. Maybe."

"Okay," I say. "I'll check back with you then."

After that, her voice disappears into static hush.

Chapter 10

Two hours later, there's still no new report about Michael's condition following his surgery. I wait another hour. Still, nothing. The medical staff at UCI Medical Center is overwhelmed, I suppose. They must be exhausted, because of the uptick in the number of COVID-19 cases, the lack of protective gear, and the pressing need to procure more ICU beds.

On a whim, I decide to drive to the hospital and try to gain entry as a visitor or, failing that, just sneak in. Bad idea, I know, but when good ideas run out, what else is left?

I leave Browny with Pa, simply because he looks so peaceful, so adorable sleeping under the bench.

The dog, I mean.

This afternoon, the sun is shining as brightly as ever, as if it never rained, but dust has caked into dry serpentine trails of mud that ornament my Escape. It's a shame, almost, to wipe it off the car—but armed with a bucket of water, my father and I attack it on all fronts, damp rags in hand, so I can take to the road.

He fingers the new scrapes on the vehicle. "Rough ride, Ash?"

"Oh, it's nothing," I say. "Don't you worry about me."

Despite my objections, Pa gives me the raincoat off his back —just in case it rains again—and tucks an envelope into the pocket, thick with ten-dollar bills.

I shake my head, refusing the money. Even though he always hands me this gift in parting, I wonder if this time, he's sensing somehow that I'm in a dire situation. Of course, I've told him nothing about my compromised bank account or my stolen identity.

"Don't say no, Ash," he says, as he bends over to kiss my cheek. "Part of it is for the expenses you had, shopping for me. As for the other part—well, consider it a loan, if you must."

I wave goodbye to him and punch the hospital's name into my GPS, only to ignore its driving instructions from the very start.

Taking an unnecessary detour through Laguna Canyon Road, I pass through the canyon and find myself coming to a stop by the Festival of Arts grounds, next door to the Laguna Playhouse. Its exterior is currently being renovated, as building is considered essential work even during the pandemic.

The Playhouse prides itself on being the oldest continuously operating theater on the West Coast. It has presented premieres featuring notable performers from Bette Davis to Harrison Ford. Why am I here? Because for me, the place holds nostalgic memories of our family, going back to the time when we regularly attended its shows.

Something here feels out of place. Maybe I'm wrong, maybe something is in place where no one expects it to be—but I can't immediately put my finger on it.

Encasing the lobby is a dramatic glass curtain. It reflects the construction workers toiling about. A quarry tile floor, clearly visible through the glass, creates a sleek, elegant interior that appears to be vacant at the moment. But this time, it's not the architecture that draws my attention—rather, it's the car parked in front.

A red 2020 Chevrolet Impala.

It looks well-cared for, with the exception of abrasions along its side, which—just as I thought—match the abrasions on my Escape. Without a doubt, this is the car that bumped me from behind and scratched against my side.

Something seems to click in my mind and, on impulse, I call my father.

His voice is heavy with concern. "Ash? Did you forget something?"

"No, don't worry. Listen, Pa, I have to ask you something. It's about your new friend."

"What about her?"

"You said, 'No more performances for Linda' and, for some reason, it makes me wonder. Is she a spectator, like you, or an actress?"

"An actress," he says. "And a fine one she is! I saw her play a brilliantly mischievous Puck in *A Midsummer's Night Dream*. When she took her final bow, I rose to my feet and couldn't stop clapping and cheering."

His glee has a strange effect on me. It makes my heart skip a beat. At last, I am coming close to identifying who means harm to me. "How does she look?"

"Linda looks the part, every time!" he says, excitedly.

"Can you describe her, Pa?"

He's silent for a moment. I imagine him pleating his forehead.

I recall the times our family would go to the theatre together. After every show, my mother would go on and on describing the costumes in more delicious detail than anyone had the appetite to absorb. About Puck she would say, with a glint in her eyes, "The arms were covered in glitter, and the legs were in green tights. Glittery makeup sparkled around the eyes. The tunic was tied with a rope around the waist. A small pair of horns peeked just a bit out of the curls of that wig. Artificial flowers and leaves, woven into it, gave the impression of a woodland sprite. "

My father just says, "A small pouch hung from the belt. It was meant for the potion Puck uses on unsuspecting humans. You know, the potion that makes them fall in love, unwittingly."

Of course, there's never anything witty about infatuation, which he proved time and time again with his woefully misguided affairs. At any rate, the costume is not what I'm curious about—what's under all that makeup is.

So, I try to stop him long enough to ask about it, but now my father won't listen, let alone take a pause.

"What more can I tell you? Sitting in the audience, I was absolutely sure the role was played by a young man," he says. "Boy, was I mistaken!"

"Pa!" I manage to say, finally. "Right now, all I want to know is this: Does she, or does she not, have sunken cheeks?"

"She does." He gasps. "How on earth did you guess?"

Just then, the glass doors pop open and—talk of the devil—Linda comes out of them. She wears no wig, no hat, no scarf. Her bald head allows me to recognize her with ease. No question, this is the woman I rescued from the waves at Pointe

Dume, the one who paid her debt of gratitude to me by emptying my bank account.

She scans the street all the way down to my Escape and, in a blink, her eyes lock with mine. I get out of my vehicle. She turns around and retreats. The glass doors swing, flashing reflections that conceal her—until coming to a close.

I take off Pa's rain jacket, shove it into the car, slam the door, and give chase.

Running around the front, I push my way through a few construction workers. Some of them are replacing the existing textured stucco on the facade with a smooth finish, others—building additions to the metal canopy. I dash forward amidst the din, accidentally knocking down their scaffolding. I go past the three ticket office windows and pull the entrance doors with all my might, trying to pry them open—only to find them locked.

I bang, bang, bang at the glass. After a while, some actor cracks the door open just enough to pop his head out.

"Where's Linda?" I ask.

The actor shrugs. "What? Who? Not here."

"I need a word with her. Let me in."

"The show has been canceled," he says, as if I asked about it. "Check online. The schedule of upcoming performances will be updated sometime in the coming days."

With that, he tries to close the door, but my foot is in it.

Enraged, I push him briskly aside and climb up the floating stairs of the grand staircase two at a time, heading towards the auditorium, where I think I see her. Her shadow seems to be slithering inside, ever so stealthily.

Gradually, my eyes adjust to the dark space sloping towards the stage. At first glance, it seems vacant, but my pounding heart tells me otherwise.

The auditorium—plush seating with red velvet cushions, punctuated with scrolled hardwood armrests—brings back fond memories. I conjure up a vision of myself down there, in the front row, wedged between my Mommy and Daddy, barely able to contain my eager anticipation for the curtains to rise.

I wish Browny were here to sniff Linda out—but at this point, I have only myself to rely on. A shiver goes down my spine. I tread, as softly as I can, along the wood railing of the upper tier, and suddenly I spot her in the lower one. Cowering in the corner of the aisle, she sneaks down the wooden stairs that lead to the bottom left exit.

I climb over the railing and onto a makeshift scaffolding, slide down a bit, and from there, hurl myself—thinking, while in flight, that I should have thought twice of doing that—and land with a splat in the aisle. Carpeting would have been nice, but there you have it. Hardwood.

I manage to roll to my knees, then dart down the stairs, where I grab her arm with a force I didn't know I possessed. With a startle, she yanks herself out of my hold and makes a sprint, first for the exit, where I block her, then for the stage.

Staggering up there, I push her into a stumble at the edge of the stage, where the two of us have a bit of a cat fight. We roll on the dusty wood floor. She's on top, then I am. She scratches my face. I shove her away, then find myself under her again. She punches me in the gut. I kick at her belly. She pulls my hair. I slap her hollow cheek.

I marvel at how strong she is, despite looking fragile. She claws at me with her nails as I gain the upper hand, but I steel myself for the pain. I pin her down, her bald head hanging over the edge.

Meanwhile, the actor rushes in. He calls out to her, "Shall I call 911?"

"Please do," I growl.

But she squeals, "No!"

"You sure, Linda?" he asks her.

"I am." She tries to catch her breath. "Do not call the police."

He repeats, "You sure?"

"Sure I'm sure. This is all just for show."

"It is?"

"Go away," she croaks. "Leave us alone."

She coughs and at once, the wind goes out of her lungs. Her resistance gone, she lies flat at my feet, no longer thrashing about.

A wave of invincibility washes over me.

Then, gloom.

My triumph, I now realize, comes with a heavy price. I've subdued her, but what makes her ill can trounce me too, in the end. This woman coughed in my face before. Two weeks ago, I thought she feigned being sick. This time, her symptoms seem to be real. And serious. I make a mental note to myself to wash my hands when I'm done with her.

Linda presses a hand against her temple and lets out a sigh, as if to release the ache that needles her. Her skin is slightly feverish to the touch, and her voice—raspy. Even she can't be that good of an actress.

In the near future, I'll have to stay away from everyone I love. I must protect them from me, from the possibility of the dreaded

Coronavirus reaching them through our closeness. I pray that they won't need my help, because I can't be there for them. My parents. My friends. Michael. Having to keep my distance, that's the best case scenario. And I don't even want to think about the worst case.

For now, let me focus on the moment. I have to make her confess. She must give the game away. "Get up," I tell her, my voice resonating with intensity. "You and I have a little case of stolen identity to sort out."

Chapter 11

Having gained the upper hand in what I consider to be round one of my battle against Linda, I support her bald head, dangling over the edge of the stage, and help her to her knees.

Meanwhile, the actor who let me in the theatre walks around the seats at the far end of the auditorium. He claps his hands as if our brawl was just a fine spectacle, as if it's all over now. But I know better. If Linda doesn't give me back what's mine—not only the money she stole from my bank account but also my identity—round two is soon to follow.

Maintaining her charade, Linda thanks him with a bow. Despite the graceful gesture, you can't be sure if it's her way to mock him. Is she in-character, playing Puck?

Once he exits, Linda gives me a signal to follow her. I slap a mask on my face, hoping it's not too late for caution.

I should have thought of it earlier, should have protected myself, because Linda is a breast cancer survivor and therefore, at high risk for contracting the deadly coronavirus. Her cough, echoing eerily in the empty auditorium, is anything but reassuring. And her figure might have been willowy in her youth, but now it is skeletal. She seems unsteady on her feet, and her smile is shaky, too.

In spite of myself, I am intrigued. How did she find her way to my father's heart? Not that it's too difficult. She was not his first affair, nor will she be the last.

My curiosity is aroused. How did Linda manage to study the way I dress, move, smile? What made her decide to play me? I saved only a small amount of money, nothing worth the trouble for committing identity theft. Didn't she fear being caught? Why take a gamble for such a meager reward?

I decide not to come to blows with her again. Instead, let me try being patient. Listen. If I do so intently, even the most clever actress can't hide behind a fake persona for long.

Together, she and I take stage exit left. We walk along a curving backstage corridor. I adjust the mask to fit tighter on my face and, with effort, control a sudden itch to rub my nose. Even through the fabric, dust tickles my nostrils. It smells of withered flowers and makeup powder.

Jolted by a sudden burst of fascination, I half-expect to rub elbows with other performers. But the long galleys where they usually prepare for the show are vacant. There is no chatter, no voices rehearsing this or that line from some script, no last-minute agitation before curtain-rise. No actors parading shamelessly in nothing but glitzy dance belts. No actresses flitting about with fluffy slippers and flapping robes that reveal more nudity than they cover.

Frosted LED globe bulbs, currently devoid of electricity, dot the top and side edges of one wall-mounted mirror after another. All the glass reflects, as Linda passes ahead of me, is a nervous tick in her hollow cheek.

Linda plops down on a vanity stool and, without losing a beat, reaches behind a freestanding vanity mirror and grabs something that's been hidden behind. A half-full bottle of

Vodka. She pours some into her mug, and her fingers tremble as she takes a long swig. Then she asks, "Want some?"

"No."

"Like my dressing room?"

I shrug. "Sure."

"It shouldn't be called that," she says. "The last thing I do in this place is put on clothes." The second gulp seems to soothe her nerves. "This, Ash darling, is where I take *me* off. I scrape away my persona, remove the extraneous layers of self that burden me."

With that, she begins to wipe off her makeup with a cotton pad, careful not to scrub the sensitive skin around the eyes. "Actually, I'm glad you came."

Which sets me back on my heels. "You are?"

"I hate being alone. In normal days, people drop in all the time—"

"In normal days," I cut in, "I would love to hear about all that—"

"I find it intoxicating when, for better or worse, people take note of me," she says, pretending not to take any note of my snide tone. "Imagine them: The director, suggesting a last-minute adjustment. An ensemble member, complaining—the poor loser—about the applause I got, which interrupted his lines. An adoring fan, bringing in a bouquet of flowers. The sound technician, testing his condom-wrapped microphone packs."

She massages some cleanser onto her skin, going around her face hairline to jawline to remove the foundation. "The theatre is the only reason why un-lubricated condoms even exist. No one ever uses them for sex."

"That's a topic for some other time," I say. "Right now, the only thing I care to discuss is why you stepped into my shoes."

"Ah. I see I made a slight mistake."

"By impersonating me?"

"No." Her chuckle sounds like anything but remorse. "By choosing the wrong bra to do so."

"Excuse me?"

Linda drains what's left in her mug and gives me a sidelong glance. "Your breasts are smaller than I thought. For playing the role of Ashley Winters, I got the wrong cup size."

I shake my head. "What you got wrong is the role."

"I like a challenge."

"Why me?"

Linda doesn't immediately answer. Instead, she leans over a wilted bouquet standing in the background behind her makeup jars. The arrangement, sent no doubt by an admirer, gives a pungent scent of decay.

It must have looked gorgeous when fresh, but now all its colors are browning. I try to imagine them the way they used to be. Vivid peach spray roses, green button pompon, pink mini carnations and yellow daisy mums, beautifully presented in a basket.

She fingers a well-worn card that hangs from one of the dry stems. "Such a giving person he is."

"Who?"

"Who else? Your darling Pa."

I'm annoyed that she's brought him into the conversation, but tell myself not to show it. "My father told me how grateful he is to you for reading his memoirs and giving him some comments—"

"In turn, the fool gave me an idea for a crime," Linda says, with a sly grin. "Not that he realized it, of course."

I pluck the card from her fingers. On it, written in my father's slanted longhand, are the words, *'You remind me of my only child.'*

To say I am not hurt would be a lie.

I turn livid. Jealous, even.

During the years of his marriage to my mother, he would bring a bouquet home on occasion, but nothing as expensive as this. At first, I tell myself that my anger is on Ma's behalf—but no. That's not it. Am I pissed at Linda because she called Pa a fool? Maybe I am. Maybe he deserves it, too—but not from the likes of her.

But above all, I'm furious at him. Why can't he think of this woman merely as his new affair, rather than as his daughter? Now, she is out to replace me in more ways than one.

Just as burning is the humiliation I suffer, realizing how she did this particular character study. Linda must have learned about me from my father's writings.

My fault, of course. By refusing to read his memoirs, I opened the door for this crook to step in. Perhaps he shared with her some old photographs of me. Perhaps they even watched old family movies together. He mistook her covert interest in me for an innocent curiosity in his literary skill.

Meanwhile, Linda takes off her black T-shirt and reaches sideways for the collapsible cloth rack, over which assorted costumes are strewn about. As she pulls out a bra from the flamboyant mishmash, the impression of her flat chest flashes across a freestanding vanity mirror. I turn my head away from the sight of her scars.

"What," she says brazenly, while filling her mug to the rim once again. "You didn't know I had a mastectomy? Your darling Pa didn't tell you?"

"He did," I admit. "What he forgot to mention is your addiction."

"Oh, that?" She clinks her mug, a bit unsteadily, against the nearly empty Vodka bottle. "Why, it's nothing. When my cancer was first diagnosed, the drink helped me face it, is all."

"I meant drugs, not alcohol. You on heroin?"

"No!"

I back off, despite my suspicion that this is her first lie, with more to follow. "Sorry. I didn't mean to pry."

Her voice turns hoarse, even worse than before, as she coughs out, "The hell you didn't."

I hold my breath and take a step back, as if that'll protect me from taking in her air.

That's when I notice a bulletin board stuck to the wall next to me. Most of it displays stage shots of wood fairies surrounding Puck, costume sketches, and snippets from Shakespeare's play, all of which must serve to inspire her, to set her in the mood before stepping onstage. But at the bottom corner of the board, there are three pages that are unrelated to the rest. They provide makeup instructions, using a facial diagram in three stages. What starts with her face, progresses—through careful application of concealer, rouge, eyeshadow, and eyeliner—into mine.

"Want to see how I do it?" she asks, mischievously now. And without waiting for my refusal, she leans into the mirror and dabs her lips with pinkish lipstick, then with gloss.

"Stop that," I say, reluctant to be swept into her game.

But then, I go for it.

I tear the mask off—precautions be dammed—and grab the jars of pressed powder. Then, I smear the darkest skin tone I can find just below my cheekbones, so from a distance greater than a couple of paces, my cheeks begin to look hollow.

With a few more touches, my lips lose their shine, and my eyebrows disappear. From the clothing rack, I pick a nylon stocking cap, nude color, and stuff my hair underneath so it's out of sight. Short of shaving it, that's the best I can do to look bald. While she is gradually becoming Ash, I am turning into Linda. In front of us, the wall mirror reflects two nearly-identical faces, each one half her, half me.

We stare at each other. She blinks.

At that moment, I think it only fitting to use Puck's lines, pinned to the board. I hop onto the vanity stool from which she has just risen. Perched on top of it as if it were a stage, I'm about to reach beyond mischief.

Linda tips her head back to look up at me. At first, she seems spellbound when I read,

If we shadows have offended,
Think but this, and all is mended,
That you have but slumber'd here
While these visions did appear.

Then she stiffens. "These are *my* lines."

"Are they? I bet I can deliver them at least as well as you. Maybe better," I boast, before pressing on.

> *Now to 'scape the serpent's tongue,*
> *We will make amends ere long;*
> *Else the Puck a liar call—*

"Enough," she growls. "Stop it!"

"Why, forgive me," I say, without bothering to hide a sarcastic note. "I thought you would have as much fun watching me steal your face as you had stealing mine."

"Fun?" she cries. Her complexion reddens to such a degree that I'm afraid she's about to lose her mind. "What the hell are you talking about? Damn you! Being Ash is no fun—"

"Tell me about it."

"And," she blurts, "it costs me dearly!"

"It does?"

Her eyes bulge out of their sockets. For a moment, I think she's going to fall apart or start screaming incoherently like a raving madwoman.

But then, out of quavering lips, she lets fly, "I'm being blackmailed for it!"

I hop off the stool. She seems close to swooning, so I fill her mug with water from a nearby sink and place it in her hand, noting the tremor.

"Linda?" I say, gently now. "Care to talk?"

Chapter 12

Linda grasps the mug, grasps it tightly in both hands. Still, it continues to rattle against her bony fingers, which makes the water spill over the rim. She hands the thing back to me and drags a fragile hand down her face as if to wipe away any trace of embarrassment. Then, she puts on the smug smile of a leading lady, talking down to the stage help. "Ash darling, can you stir in some honey?"

Out of pity, I play along. I ask where it can be found.

From her vanity stool, Linda points at a small jar that stands between an ashtray and her Vodka bottle. "Being a renowned actress, I must keep my vocal cords in tiptop shape, you know."

I pour a generous amount of honey into the mug, stir it briskly, and put it to her lips. She takes a sip, then complains it has no flavor and that nothing has any taste lately.

I heard somewhere that a new loss of taste or smell is one of the symptoms of coronavirus, which makes me eager to bolt out of her presence. But if I do so, I'll never learn why she stole my identity and who else knows about it, knows enough to demand something more out of her.

"So, you're being blackmailed?" I ask, holding myself back from asking the obvious, "By whom?"

Her shoulders sag as she hangs her head down, sighs. "Who would have guessed a little stunt—like putting on your face and swaying my hips the way you do—would end up this badly?"

I click my tongue, mockingly. "Indeed. Who could have guessed."

"What a bummer." Linda gets up and paces to and fro, clearly agitated. She reaches for a cigarette box and flips the top open. "Not my fault, of course."

"Of course not."

"I was dared to do it. I was led to believe that your bank account had tens of thousands of dollars for the taking, and who could pull it off better than me?"

At the mention of this ridiculously high estimate of my savings, I'm torn between wanting to burst out in laughter and dying to cry. Either way, I'm puzzled. "How could anyone know how much money I have? I thought such information is supposed to be private!"

Linda struts around me, stopping only long enough to light a cigarette, then angles it between her nicotine-stained fingers this way and that. She lets time pass, perhaps to consider how much detail she's ready to reveal.

"This guy, he's a bank employee," she says, at last. "At the time, I thought he was the manager. He said he was, anyway. What's more, he knew all about my loan application, promised to approve it, too—but said he had to pull some strings first, because my income had fluctuated this year from one month to another. Unfortunately, I could present no proof of what I could earn in the future, except for fame, which is a fickle thing—"

"This guy, does he have a name?"

"Oleg. Oleg Kuznetsov." Linda pleats her brow, clearly annoyed that I've interrupted her, but makes no mention of it for now. "When I first met him, the Irvine branch was already closed for the day, but he let me in. Perhaps he saw how distraught I was. Or else, he recognized me. As an actress, I'd like to believe that."

"So, what was your first impression?"

"Right away, I wondered how a heavy-handed man like him, with such a loaded accent, managed to rise to a position of authority at Wells Fargo."

"Accent? What kind?"

"Russian. With a name like that, what did you expect?"

I shrug, and Linda looks at the ceiling, as if to find her train of thought up there. She takes a long drag of her Camel, then lets out a puff of smoke. "I don't like your silly questions. Don't try to confuse me, Ash darling, or this conversation is over."

"Sorry."

"Anyway, where was I? Oh yes. Something seemed a bit off about him, but I told myself that diversity at a workplace is a good thing. So what if he's a foreigner? So what if he has the physique of a gorilla? An imposing presence can be an asset for a man's career. And sometimes life is stranger than fiction, right? In the theatre, no director would cast a guy with those fat sausage fingers to play a white-collar character, let alone a bank manager—but in real life, you never know, do you?"

"So, you decided to put your trust in him."

"I did. Can you imagine my shock when I discovered—the day after emptying your account—that he's part of the bank's cleaning crew?"

"What?"

"You heard right. In hindsight, I see it now all too clearly. Everything Oleg knew about me must have come from sifting through my loan application papers. Maybe he found them atop a stack of papers on the manager's desk or in his wastebasket."

In a sudden fury, Linda kicks her own stool, which makes it topple over. "You would think that with my experience in show business, I wouldn't be fooled by the performance of a lesser actor. Wrong! Oh why, why, why did I blind myself to the truth?"

"Perhaps you wanted to believe him."

"I did. It's not that he managed to convince me that he was who he claimed he was. I convinced myself."

"So you had no clue—"

"None." She scratches her bald head. "On second thought, that's not exactly true. I did get an anonymous note warning me about Oleg, about his conduct with women. But I didn't care about that. I was lonely. I needed attention, and his was better than nothing—or so I thought."

She shakes her head, sniffs. "What's more, I was desperate. I could no longer afford to buy gas for my car. Medical bills were piling up with no end in sight. I had to get that loan or, failing that, some money—no matter where it came from."

Exasperated, I snap. "Where it came from was the wrong place. My pocket."

"Sorry, darling," she says, but I doubt she means it. "Of course, I could have sold my Impala—but hated the thought of it. I needed to keep up appearances."

"I understand," I say, just to keep her talking.

Linda extinguishes the cigarette butt. "Anyway, I waited anxiously for being approved and, at the same time, started spending time with Oleg."

"Your place or his?"

"Neither. I would meet him for coffee at Cafe De Mama, or he would drive me to Huntington Beach and we would walk along the pier."

"Oh, how lovely."

She seems not to catch my acidic tone. "It does sound that way, doesn't it? Anyway, Oleg is a closet drunkard, like me. Somehow, it felt good to share a bottle of Vodka in someone's company—even his—especially since he would pay for it. Beyond that, incredible as it may sound, there was nothing intimate."

I raise an eyebrow, because her claim of a purely platonic affair sounds hollow. It sounds like a lie.

Linda is quick to explain. "Don't you see? Because I have no breasts, he treated me like damaged goods, which is why he never laid hands on me like he did other girls."

"Now that's a relief," I mutter, under my breath.

She lights up another Camel and glares at me. "But it doesn't mean he found no other uses for what I can do. Quite the contrary."

"And what was it, exactly, that he had in mind?"

"Oleg dared me to cash your savings. He said we could split the dough, but most of it would go to me. If I played it right, he said, no one at the bank would even notice. He would make sure of that, somehow. So whether or not my loan was approved, I would be taken care of."

I wish there was more Vodka to keep her talking. Failing that, I fill her mug with more water and mix it with more honey.

Linda licks her lips, greedily. "Oleg said he would drive me to a Wells Fargo branch in any other town, because here in Irvine, some of the clerks might have been friends with you. Of course, without your driver's license there was no point at all to his plan, no matter the location, and I told him so. He said he knew your address—"

"What?"

"You lived on UCI campus, or so he said. He was willing to break in while you were asleep to get all the necessary ID cards from your purse. No way, I said. Certain limits should not be crossed, and I drew the line at burglary. So Oleg said never mind, he was just joking."

Her story is devolving into a train wreck, whether she knows it or not. The only saving grace in it is that so far, it seems that this guy didn't know I'd moved to LA. I draw in a deep breath and tell myself to relax, which is easier said than done.

"His next idea was to forge the damn cards." Linda takes a sip. "Again, I refused."

Having taken a lot of courses in product design, I can appreciate the technical difficulty of selecting the right card stock and ink, let alone designing a perfect seal stamp. "It takes talent to forge—"

"It takes talent to act," she cuts in. "And who better than me?"

"Indeed," I say. "No one."

"When Oleg came up with the idea of playing you, I was intrigued."

"Where did you find the chutzpah to actually go ahead with it?"

Linda bares her teeth in a sly smile. "Chutzpah was never the issue—but what I lacked, at first, was inspiration."

"What does that mean?"

Linda taps the filter tip, flicking the ember into the ashtray. Another ring of smoke sails into the air. "Not knowing much about you, there was no way for me to do a proper character study. So I said goodbye to Oleg, determined not to see him again. But then, guess what? That very night, after curtain fall, the old fool came along."

Realizing who she's talking about, I clench my teeth.

"Ah, he so adored my Puck! My performance, he said, was so captivating, so brilliantly mischievous! He begged me to meet him, sent flowers to my dressing room, along with a touchingly written card. By his signature, I realized who he was. Your darling Pa."

I swallow the hurt and, with a tone as even as I can produce, say, "So let me see if I get it, Linda. You thought that meeting my Pa was somehow a sign from heaven that you should go along with a crime."

Linda claps her hands. "Exactly! As soon as your father showed me your picture, which he always carries in his wallet, and told me those cute family stories, saying how proud he was of you, I had a good handle on the role. All my doubts vanished, as did the occasional dread."

"Dread?" I echo.

She wipes some sweat from her brow. "I no longer feared that someone might catch me redhanded when I get my hands on the dough, or that news of a once-famous star, driven to theft because of a declining career, would hit the papers. That, in itself, used to torture me. It stole sleep from my eyes—even more so than the prospect of being thrown in prison."

I can't help wondering, out loud, "And what made you so sure you could pull it off?"

Linda waves a hand at me and reaches over to the wig holder, which I haven't noticed earlier: a heavy duty canvas-covered mannequin head with no facial features, set upon a round stand made of wood. With a swift motion, she removes the wig from it.

"Ash darling, you may think that acting is merely pretense," she says, looking at me down her nose. "That's a common mistake. Acting is all about unearthing an inner truth about the character and finding a way to bring it to the surface. For me, it wasn't enough to slap a hairy thing over my head or smear my lips with gloss. I had to pull you—all of you, everything that happened to you in the past, everything you wish to become in the future—down into my soul."

Who does Linda think she is? I bite my lips, praying she's merely delusional, hoping she doesn't know everything that happened to me, because no strangers should be in on my secret. Certainly, my father didn't tell her about it, about my rape. Or did he?

Meanwhile, she clicks a light switch. Frosted LED globe bulbs shine across the top and side edges of her wall-mounted mirror. She also turns on the light of the freestanding vanity mirror, then fits the wig on her head. It makes her seem both punky and gorgeous. I hate to say she looks like me.

The hairstyle is identical to mine, down to the layered wisps of hair around the neck, which Ma often describes as an explosion in a noodle factory. But that's not what is so striking to me—rather, it's the glint in Linda's eyes, reflected in both mirrors. It says, I am Ashley Winters, I and no other! And who the hell are you?

In a blink, I feel depleted.

I pull the nylon stocking cap off my head and shake my curls free, to remind myself that between the two of us, I am the real Ash, her so-called *inner truth* be damned.

"You know, I did a dress rehearsal for Oleg." Linda adjusts the wig, then wraps a curl around her finger as playfully as I often do. "And that, Ash darling, was the only time I saw him aroused."

"Not a pretty sight, I bet."

"Plain ugly." She shakes her head. "Afterwards, I felt like calling the whole thing off. But I didn't. Not only because of the money. At that point, I couldn't give up playing the role. I simply fell in love with it. I had to be you."

"Which reminds me." I harden my voice to let her know I mean business. "I need my identity back."

"Huh, I bet you do."

"Give me back what's mine."

Linda pretends not to understand. "What?"

"My ID cards."

She shrugs. "I don't have them."

"What?"

"I threw them away."

And just as I struggle with the urge to wring out the neck of this liar, some distant ramble makes me freeze. It comes from the direction of the auditorium.

At first, I think it must be the skinny actor who let me in, as no one else but him seemed to be hanging around. But when the stage sighs, all of a sudden, under a heavy footfall, I realize it can't be a light-footed guy.

Startled, Linda clasps my arm, which makes my heart skip a beat, and the breath flutters in her throat—but she can't hold it for long. She coughs.

For a moment, nothing. Just a hissing hush.

I perk my ears.

After a long while, the stage creaks again under someone's weight.

Linda hisses, "What's *he* doing here?"

And I whisper, "Who?"

She rises unsteadily to her tiptoes, so her pumps won't clink against the floor, and looks nervously left and right, as if to figure out her next move. "Let's hide."

At once, those footsteps rock the place again. By the thumping sound, they exit stage left, then go along the curving backstage corridor—just the way we've come in here, to her dressing room. Linda reaches over to one switch, then another, and cuts off electricity. The bulbs of both mirrors go dark.

Of one thing I'm sure: Whoever he is, this sudden murkiness will not stop him. He can blindly sniff her out by her smoky scent alone. And by her shiver, she knows it, too.

Even before my eyes fully adjust to the shadows, I detect a huge silhouette coming down the dim galley. A faint ray, spilling in from a distant half-open back door, falls askew on his hand. At the sight of his fat sausage fingers, Linda bends over her stomach as if it's tied in knots.

She knows who it is, and so do I.

Chapter 13

I don't know for sure if Linda is infectious, but her anxiety certainly is. I tell myself to snap out of it. She's the one Oleg intends to blackmail, not me. True, he did dare her to steal my money, but—as far as I know—he poses no danger to my life. After all, my bank account is empty. I have nothing left to offer. So why is her fear gripping me, too?

On second thought, there is still room for worry. Linda and I have just exchanged appearances, so he may very well mistake me for her. With the dark makeup I've smeared under my cheekbones, my cheeks look sunken, just like hers. I've dusted off my eyebrows and dulled the shine of my lips. By now, my clothes are impregnated with her cigarette smoke. I glance at my reflection. Why, my own mother wouldn't recognize me!

And as for Linda, she's applied pink lipstick with gloss and penciled the shape of my eyebrows, ever so perfectly. Her wig is cut in the same style as my hair. What's more, her C-cup bra, worn across that flat chest of hers, makes a point of being incredibly curvaceous.

Unfortunately, this moment is a stage call. There is no time for a do-over. The show must go on.

Now facing us, Oleg stops in his tracks and shifts his gaze from her to me and back again, in obvious confusion. He looks just the way Linda has described him, down to his fat sausage fingers. But she's forgotten to mention his tattoo: a scaly snake slithering around his triceps, then in and out of the serpentine letters inked above his elbow. *Voola*.

The tattoo starts at the back of his thick neck, disappears under the frayed collar of his shirt, and slips out the sleeve over his arm. There, it surrounds the reddish track marks, probably caused by repeated heroin injections, masking them away.

His armpits reek of sour sweat, but that's not what startles me—his voice does.

"Vill the real Miss Vinters step forward?" he asks, as if he were the host of some TV gameshow, as if the answer will not bear any harrowing consequences.

Painfully etched into my memory, this is the voice of the man whose face I've had trouble recalling, ever since I woke up, months ago, from my coma. I've been dreading the moment of coming into his presence again, despite being committed to find him and avenge myself.

This is the thug who raped me.

I shudder.

The scene is seared into my mind. It traps me before I can breathe, before I can extricate myself from the memory. It all started when someone pulled hard at my scarf. I thought he might strangle me with it. Instead, he stuffed it down my throat, so I couldn't even cry for help.

How can I forget? The attacker kicked my legs to spread them apart and pinned me under his weight. The first blow stunned me. Blood started gushing down my brow. I struggled. I even tried to scratch out the white of his eye. Marbled with tortuous veins—just the way it looks at me now—that horrific eye was the only thing I could see before passing out.

A bead of sweat trickles down my spine. Right now, I feel quite silly under the war-paint that covers my face—but luckily, it works. Oleg seems not to recognize me for who I am. Instead, he stares at Linda, who is doing her Ashley impersonation. Which gives me a moment to rehash what I've learned about their so-called friendship.

She did a dress rehearsal before, playing me for him. I can only imagine how she swayed her hips and batted her false eyelashes, ever so innocently, in preparation for stealing my identity. According to her, it aroused him. Only now do I understand why.

In his sick mind, beating me unconscious was not an unpleasant memory: my weakness, his power. I hope he didn't try to replicate that thrill. I hope he didn't molest her, too.

And if he did, I bet she would deny it.

Right now, Linda just stands there, her back to the wall, her arms hanging limp. Paralyzed.

"Vell, there," Oleg tells her, in his heavy Russian accent. "It's been quite a vile since the last time I saw you, vat's your name."

"Ashley," she says, managing somehow to stay in-character. "And don't you forget the sound of it."

He licks his fat lips, his tongue hanging over the unshaven whiskers.

"Ah-huh," he growls. "Ashley."

"That name," she says, "is the last thing you'll ever hear." And with a sudden jerk, she pulls out a Kimber Micro 9mm pistol from somewhere behind her back and points it at his head.

Despite her swagger, Linda can't control the thing. It begins rattling in her grasp.

Oleg must sense that she's all show and no action. He takes a cautious step forward. In a minute, he'll snatch it from her unsteady fingers. So what choice do I have? I grab it before he does.

She crumples to the floor, like a pile of bones. I turn swiftly to him. "You," I say. "Step back."

My voice sounds surprisingly steely. He obeys—but bends his knee slightly as if in preparation for a sprint.

In a snap, I aim the pistol at the ceiling, pull the trigger, and then—*boom!*—a warning shot rings out. At once, Oleg covers his ears in fright and, with a thwack, falls to his knees before me.

"You mean business, yes, yes, I see zat very vell, Linda." He gulps. "But, but vee are partners!"

"Are we?" I bring the barrel next to my lips and with a little puff, blow off smoke. "I don't know what to think about a partner who tries to blackmail me."

"Vat blackmail?" he cries, raising his hands in defeat. "Forget it, Linda! Vee planned perfect crime—"

"Out, out, out! If you're still here by the count of three, I'll blow your brains out."

"Vy?" His eyes bulge in disbelief. "You are good, very good at vat you do, Linda. Getting into Miss Vinters' account vas like nothing for you. And for us, it vas only the beginning!"

Although I have a lot of questions in my mind about the identity theft scheme and how he plans to roll out more of it in the future, I'm getting tired of this talk, and especially of playing her. Being Linda has been fun for a bit, but now it's troublesome. It sucks who I am right out of my skin.

Ignoring everything he says, I count, "One."

He starts creeping away on all fours faster than I thought possible. "But—"

"Two—"

He crawls down the long galley on all fours and, once at a safe distance, bolts out. His footfalls are now echoing out in the auditorium.

I follow him all the way down to the lobby. And as I count, "Three," the theater entrance doors slam to a close, and he's gone.

Meanwhile, Linda drags her feet behind me. I glance at her over my shoulder. She removes her hand from her mouth, no longer muffling the chatter of her teeth. The pink lipstick has smudged unevenly under her nose and all around her chin.

She shakes her head. "Why?"

"Why what?"

"You had the chance to finish him off once and for all. Why the hell didn't you? Ash darling, this is a moment to regret."

"Linda darling," I say, using the same dejected tone, "the moment you threw my ID cards away is the one to regret. You better find them for me."

"Fine." She gives me a tentative nod. "I'll look for them."

"Hand them over by tomorrow."

"I'll do my best."

"And if you don't," I say, "I'll report you to the police."

Linda takes a step back. "No need to use threats—"

"No need, once you do your part. Just so you know, they're already investigating the case and will be thrilled when I point them to you as the principal suspect."

I go back to her dressing room and drop her pistol next to the ashtray. In a snap, the wind goes out of me. She's right. What was I thinking? I should've killed him—or, failing that, I should've called 911, so they would have him arrested, not to mention compare his DNA to the traces left inside of me.

"My mistake," I admit. "But I don't need someone like you to dole out guilt. I am generating that masterfully on my own."

Ready to leave, I stand in the lobby next to her and watch through the glass as life goes on out there. Construction workers come down from the scaffolding, pack their tools next the front facade, leave. It's the end of a workday. Couples pass across the street, holding hands. It's the beginning of a lovely midsummer evening.

I check my cellphone and notice a missed call from UCI Medical. It must have vibrated while my shot rang out. I call back, and the receptionist tells me the good news. Michael is now in recovery, the bullet has been successfully extracted from his shoulder, and he's doing as well as can be expected.

I ask, "Can I talk to him?"

"Just a minute."

By the subtle click, she's transferred the call. A moment later, I hear him. "Ash?"

"Oh, Michael! I'm so glad to hear you! How d'you feel?"

"Don't worry about me, sweetheart," Michael says, his voice a bit groggy. "Where are you? I hear some echo."

"In the lobby of a theatre."

"Really? You've been to a play?" He sounds downright jealous. "Without me?"

Some play this was. "I'll tell you all about it when we meet. All I can say now is that the casting was lousy."

He's silent for a moment.

"Michael?" I whisper. "All I can say is I love you."

"Don't say anything more," he says, "till you are in my arms."

"All right," I say, playfully. "My lips are sealed."

"Are you alright, sweetheart? I hear someone wheezing—"

"Don't worry, Michael," I say, distancing myself a few more paces from Linda. Thanks to her, I'll have to self-quarantine, again. "It isn't me."

After the call ends, I mark the date—two weeks from now—on my cellphone's calendar. Even if he's released from the hospital before then, I'll have to keep myself away for his sake. In his present condition, he is vulnerable to infection.

Oh, I can't wait. I long for him so.

Chapter 14

I head over to my Escape. On one side of me, storefronts. Most of them are boarded up for fear of looting. Which one of them used to sell ceramics? Which one—oil paintings? Artistic jewelry? Statuettes? At this point, hard to tell.

On the other side of me, a cloudy sunset. Partially blocked by the silhouette of the theatre, the sun is descending through haze to meet its reflection on the horizon. As the last glimmer starts dimming out, a chill goes down my spine. If not for the sudden pang of hunger, I would call it a night.

In just over two weeks, it's my twenty-second birthday. No reason to celebrate. I feel way older than that.

This is a new world. A world where you can never be sure what to believe; where a pandemic is called a hoax, which allows it to spread unabated; where, in the face of a rising death toll, the promise of a vaccine is being dangled without any scientific basis whatsoever by politicians who'll do just about anything to remain in power; where you better stay more than a breath away from crowds; where you must protect yourself from a hug, a handshake can be dangerous, and a kiss can kill.

I rub a bit of sanitizer on my hands. The provisions I packed with me—bottled water and a few sandwiches—are long gone. I reach over to the back of the car and retrieve the shiny tin can Ma gave me this morning. I open the lid, and a metallic bottom glares up at me. My stomach growls. I blame it on my lack of self-discipline. No more cookies. Just a few crumbs and a lone chocolate chip rolling noisily about, bumping against its mirror image.

Checking my cellphone, I notice several text messages from Rita. I call her, and she gets straight to the point. "Did you file a police report?"

I roll my eyes. "I did, but so far the case seems hopeless. I heard nothing from them. Didn't you tell me they ran the bank surveillance image of that woman through face recognition technology and came up empty?"

"This technology is known to have some inaccuracies," she admits. "It uses biometrics—such as the distance between the eyes and from the forehead to the chin—to come up with a formula, called a *facial signature*. This, then, is compared to a database of known faces. But mistakes do happen."

"Why?"

"Well, mistakes can be caused by bias, by misinformation—"

"Or by fooling the eye," I say.

"Fooling the eye?" she echoes. "How?"

"A thick layer of cosmetics might do the trick."

Rita chuckles, but I remain serious. No one at the bank caught Linda when she painted her face to look like mine. Oleg himself was deceived. Equally bewildering, he could not identify me when I painted my face to look like hers. Facial recognition technology is as prone to error as the eye of a human.

If my parents were present in her dressing room, would they have recognized me? Would Michael? I don't really know. The only one I trust not to be fooled is the dog.

"Oh well." I wave my hand. "There's no more money in my account. I can simply close it and forget the whole thing."

"Someone's got your medical insurance," Rita says. "These days, you never know when you'll need it."

"I happened to know who that someone is."

She gasps. "What?"

"Her name," I say, "is Linda Leigh."

"When did you figure it out?"

"Just about an hour ago."

Rita pleats her brow. "I think I've heard that name. Isn't she an actress?"

"Yes. Also, a breast cancer survivor—"

"Oh my!" Rita cries. "All the more reason to report her! If you don't, she'll have you on the hook, going forward, for her chemo and radiation treatments—"

"I don't think she will. We talked. She knows I know."

"Well, did you get your ID cards back from her?"

"Well, not yet—"

"Then, it's going to be a big mess to sort out later."

"Linda told me she threw the cards away."

"And you believed her?"

"No, but what choice do I have? I can't force her to give back what she doesn't have. I made her promise to find them."

Without missing a beat, Rita says, "She lied."

"Yes," I say. "She probably did."

"With your driver's license in hand, this woman can go to the DMV and declare she now lives at a new address. She can go to the post office and get your mail redirected. All the medical insurance statements would go to her. You won't even know that you owe money for her hospitalization and treatments until who knows when."

With a sigh, I relent. "Fine, Rita. You convinced me."

I get out of the car and rush back. The theatre is already dark. No one answers when I knock on the glass door. The realization that Rita is right dawns on me, hard. My driver's license and medical insurance card are in Linda's hands, which leaves me with no choice but to act now. On second thought, Linda knows I'll report her to the police tomorrow morning. Not much can happen between now and then, so what's the harm in waiting?

Thanks to Pa's generosity, I can afford dining out. These days, it's not as carefree as it used to be. The Centers for Disease Control and Prevention now report an increased risk for contracting the virus in restaurants, because wearing a mask while shopping is doable, not so while eating and drinking.

I drive to Los Olivos Marketplace. My favorite kebab shop is called—what else?—*The Kebab Shop*. To deal with the latest restrictions on restaurants, they now offer a curbside pickup. In previous visits, I had falafels. Tonight I have a craving for the flatbread wrap.

The bread is thin and soft, tightly wrapped around the carved chicken and pickled onions, and it has a slightly charred flavor. I dip it in the garlic yogurt and the cilantro sauce, then sink my teeth in. Ah, heaven! The first bite works wonders to quell the pang of hunger and clear my mind. By the time I guzzle the last of the crispy fries, I know my next step.

First and foremost, I must make sure that I'm not on the hook for Linda's medical procedures. I sift through the shopping bag Ma gave me this morning. It is overflowing with all kinds of envelopes—most of them junk mail—forwarded to her from my previous address. I find only three letters of interest.

The first is a letter from Clearwater, Florida. It's from Timmy, the boy I tutored while spending a semester break there. He sends me a picture of his turtle, winding its way toward the water's edge. His dream, he writes, is visiting the Galapagos Islands one day, when it's safe to fly.

The second is a letter from India. It's from Karishma, my dear friend who used to work at Annapoorna Indian Cuisine, here in Irvine. When the pandemic hit, buffet-style dining went out of favor. Then came the layoffs. Out of work, she traveled to her place of birth and ended up staying there. Now, she sends me pictures of the village people, wearing colorful fabric masks that she has sewed for them with her own hands.

And the third letter—well, the third one is from my health insurance. It contains a medical bill. Right away, something about it stinks to high heaven.

My previous bills would list procedures taken to keep me alive, dating back to the time I was in a coma. But no, that's not what's in this bill. I recall that Linda had a mastectomy recently. With my own eyes, I saw the scars on her flat breast. So I prepare myself for seeing a phony charge for that procedure. But no, that's not it, either. The procedure I'm being billed for—get this!—is a vasectomy.

What?

I rub my eyes, look at it again, laugh out loud.

This is clearly a mistake. It should be the easiest thing in the world to prove wrong. First thing, tomorrow morning.

Utterly exhausted, I park for the night at UCI campus, in a secluded spot shaded by trees. Through the branches, I have a partial view of the apartment I used to rent just before the pandemic hit. Someone else lives there now. Someone else has just turned off the light.

I snuggle down in my sleeping bag. The moonlit scene, this dreamy image of my past, seems both familiar and alien to me now. I close my eyes and, despite the lack of certainty in my future, feel as if in the end, everything will be all right. Somehow.

At dawn, I take a second look at the bill, studying it in detail, starting with the doctor's name—Dr. Leo Cohen—which suddenly, rings a bell. It is identical to the name of my mother's neighbor, the one who committed suicide.

I call her. "Morning, Ma. Did I wake you?"

I hear her swallowing a yawn. She must be rolling out of bed and into a leap of intuition. "Ashley? What happened? Why are you calling so early? You in some kind of trouble?"

"No, Ma," I say, as soothingly as I can. "Everything is just fine. Listen, I have a question for you. It's about your neighbor, Dr. Cohen."

"Oh , the poor soul. May he rest in peace."

"I forget, where was his office?"

"Why, you have some skin problem?"

"No, but—"

"I see, you don't want to tell me. I get it. Everything is a big secret with you, Ashley." She sighs. "Oh well, I can recommend someone else in the same office. It's Beach Cities Dermatology, Medical Center of Irvine. Wait a minute, let me find the exact address."

"I can find it myself," I say. "You know, I'm looking at this medical bill—"

"For you?"

"No," I lie, hoping to stop her from this relentless meddling, or at least slow it down just a bit. "For a friend. You don't know him."

"Oh, really?" There is a new note of enthusiasm in her voice. "You have a new boyfriend now? Someone I might like, for a change?"

"Please, Ma! Can you stop?"

"Fine, I won't say another word," she mutters, only to break her promise on the spot. "So? What about that bill?"

"Well, it was issued by a doctor by the same name and the same credentials—but practicing at a different address."

"Where, exactly?"

"In Los Angeles."

"Must be someone else, then," she says. "Cohen is a common name, after all."

"Yes. It is."

This dermatologist claims to have performed a vasectomy. I spare her this inexplicable little detail because it'll send her into a wild tailspin. She'll wonder if my new boyfriend, who doesn't even exist, went through some weird sex change operation. Perhaps she'll even retract her objection to Michael, my love.

Oh, I can only wish.

For me, this bill offers the first hint of a much larger scam. I'm beginning to sense that this is more than some petty crime concocted by a thug and executed by a has-been actress. Perhaps I am not the only medical insurance beneficiary to become a victim of this scam. This is big. Can I get my hands around it?

Chapter 15

I try to contact the dermatology clinic, hoping to prove that I was never treated by anyone there for anything, let alone a vasectomy. Why would they even offer such a procedure? It is more than skin deep, obviously outside the scope of their medical specialty. Why would they even offer the procedure to a female patient? Why me? Clear my record, I say, and cancel the nonsensical charge. An apology for the mix-up would be nice, too.

I leave a message on the answering machine. Hours later, it remains unanswered. I can't say I'm surprised.

So I hit the road, determined to get to LA and find that clinic before the end of the business day. Can you blame me for blowing off my earlier decision to lay low? Self-quarantine is a tedious thing. I've done it before. I'm tired of it now. Fuming, I puff my cheeks. I feel like I'm burning. Maybe it's rage. Maybe fever. I have a devious urge to breathe on this Dr. Cohen character so he, too, catches fire.

Just kidding.

This used to be rush hour—or more precisely, a stretch of four long hours or even more, starting at two in the afternoon, during which you would be stuck in bumper-to-bumper traffic. But now, the drive is surprisingly smooth. Boring, even. Because of the stay-at-home directive, there are few cars on the 405 highway. From time to time, a gray van appears in the rearview mirror, somewhere in the far distance. A couple of refrigerator trucks trundle in front.

I turn on the car radio, flip between this station and that, hoping to plunge myself into the clamor of news reports. As long as I do that, the loneliness sending its cold, creepy fingers toward my heart will be held at bay. In the presence of a good tale, it will go away.

I flip to another radio station. Nothing holds my interest for long. But then, as I enter the city and pass through Skid Row, a story comes on the air that quickens my pulse. It's about the 2010 Medicaid fraud case, committed by a gang called *The Armenian Power*.

Wait, wait! I remember this story. The other day, I even read it out loud for my dad. The leaders of this organized crime group, based in New York and Los Angeles, were eventually caught. I suppose they're rotting in jail. Still, I wonder if the idea of their scam could has propagated, somehow, to the outside world. If it did, then a new version of that fraud is now claiming new victims.

I may be one of them.

Knowing that Pa loves mafia stories of any kind, I call him. "Pa, remember *The Armenian Power*? Their fraud case is being told right now on the radio. Want to hear?"

By the slight rustle, I figure he's just set aside his newspaper. "Sure do!"

We listen to the radio together, which makes the physical distance that grows between us seem to shrink.

"The scammers!" he chuckles. "Can you believe it?"

I force out a laugh. "Funny, right?"

But then, I cringe. By hearing how the fraud unfolded in the past, I begin to see how in the future, my own stolen identity can be used in combination with false medical claims.

Ten years ago, the scammers rented mailboxes from a private company which, unlike the post office, gave the appearance of real street addresses, while leaving a smaller paper trail.

Using these misleading addresses, the scammers registered fake, non-existent clinics with the state—and later, with the federal government—as medical providers.

Meanwhile, they stole doctors' identities, finding most of the information—such as dates of birth and medical licensing—on public websites for doctors. Then, they matched this data with Social Security numbers, available for purchase on the black market.

As for Medicare beneficiaries, the scammers often called senior citizens, pretending to represent Medicare, and simply asked for their personal data.

At hearing this, Pa gasps. "Ha! I got such a call, just the other day!"

"What?" Suddenly, I remember his so-called friend Linda. Behind his back, she called him an old fool. I pray he didn't do anything that might prove her right.

"Turn off the radio," Pa says. "I've heard enough."

I'm about to pull out my hair in frustration—but manage, somehow, to keep a lid on it. "So, tell me exactly what happened."

"The caller was nice, I mean, she had a lovely voice."

"Did you recognize her?"

There is some unease in his silence. Then, "No," he says, but his tone is tentative. "Not really."

"Sounds like a definite maybe to me."

He doesn't dispute it. "Anyway, she told me that according to the Contact Tracing system, I'm likely to have been in close proximity to someone who tested positive for the virus."

At once, guilt kicks in. Perhaps, by coming to visit Pa, I carried the disease to him? "Did she tell you who that person was?"

"No. I asked, but she said it's confidential."

"Okay. Then what?"

"Then, she said I should be tested within the next seventy-four hours for COVID-19. She asked for my address so she can send me a testing kit. I thought that was generous."

"So, you gave her your address?"

"I did. Was that the wrong thing to do?"

Over his question, I ask, "Was that all this woman wanted?"

"No, she also asked for a credit card so she could finalize my purchase."

"What?"

"That's exactly what I said! I asked her, 'What purchase? I thought the test was at no cost to me?' and she laughed. She said, 'No, nothing is free, don't you know that? There is a one-time fee of sixty dollars for the kit and test results, and would you please read the card number to me, I'm ready when you are.'"

I hesitate to ask, "So, did you?"

"Well no, I said with my pension I can't afford it, and these days I'm all alone anyway, so even in the worst case, I pose no danger to anyone."

"Was that the end of it?"

"No. She insisted that testing is necessary, so I did what I do best: play stubborn. I said that if my time comes, so be it, and thank you but no, thank you. She said there are penalties for not complying, which made me gulp. At last, she offered to waive the charges and instead, bill Medicare, which is something she's prepared to do for no one else but me, if I give my Social Security number—"

I let out a gasp. "Oh my!"

"What, you think I'm a fool?"

"No, Pa, I don't, but—"

"This is how clever I am: I hung up."

By now, I've turned into the street where the dermatology clinic is supposed to be. I sweep my eyes across the facades, looking for a medical building. So far, nothing looks like one. I pass one empty storefront after another. The search looks increasingly pointless, but by the street numbers, I know I'm getting closer.

"Ash?" Pa says. "You're so silent. Is it something I said?"

"Oh, no, Pa! I'm just looking around for a place to park," I say. "Can we talk later?"

"Sure, Ash. Love you."

"Love you too, Pa."

A bark is heard in the background, which makes my heart ache. "And I miss Browny so much. Give him a big hug for me."

*

I park and get out, just as a gray van pulls to the curb on the opposite side. The evening breeze pushes against me as I walk down Main Street. I pass under a broken street lamp, which makes me thankful that I've arrived before nightfall. This used to be a fun place to shop—but now, I wouldn't like to find myself here after dark.

The first store sign—Cap & Hat Imports—has its 'C' dangling on a nail, twisting this way and that with every gust of wind. Next to it, The Dish Factory has a *Store Closing Sale* sign. The store after that is boarded up, with some junk piled in front. The next one, across a side street, is just coming into view.

I hop over the three steps leading up to the store. The door is locked. I back down. A reflection of myself is slowing to a standstill as I approach the store window. Mashing my nose into it, I try to get a glimpse through the murky surface.

The place looks deserted, not a single person in sight. Cardboard boxes are strewn across the floor, some with their flaps hanging open, partially filled with some stuff. One box is standing on its side, next to a heap of party poppers. Another box is folded, leaning flatly against the back wall. Balloons and confetti litter the entire floor. This place is no clinic. It is a party supply store gone broke.

Just in case I've missed anyone in the shadowy corners, I go up again and knock on the door. Above the handle, there is a mail slot. Its mouth is crammed solid with papers, as if unable to either swallow or spit them out.

I glance left and right, making sure no one sees me pulling out some of the envelopes. They are addressed to the same dermatology clinic I've been hoping to find. A non-existent one.

I tear open a few of the envelopes. Reading the letters, I realize I should call the police at once. But first, I take snapshots of several letters. The camera flash startles me. I glance over my shoulder, my breath catching in my thudding chest. The street looks empty still, but I feel as if I'm being watched. Must be just my imagination.

I punch 911 and in a hurried voice, whisper, "I want to report a massive insurance fraud."

The man at the other end takes my name, then says, "How do you know about it?"

"I am one of its victims."

"And you are?"

"Ashley Winters."

"Okay. Tell me what you know."

"It seems that a phony clinic—perhaps one of many—has been established to bill insurance companies hundreds of thousands of dollars in false claims."

"For what, exactly?"

"For procedures that no patient ever received and no doctor ever performed."

"Do you have any proof?"

"I do," I say. "I have snapshots of complaints sent to this clinic. Let me text them to you."

"Okay," he says, once I send him what I have. "You'll hear from us."

I know I should leave this place. The sooner the better. But first, I'm tempted to tell Rita I have a scoop for her. She'll be thrilled to investigate it. Besides, her police friend may be able to follow up on the fraud case. I need all the help I can get.

From out of nowhere, a smell of sweat wafts in the air.

I make the mistake to ignore it until after I text Rita the snapshots. Which is when I feel a tap, a nagging tap on my shoulder. In the glass, behind my mirror image, are the reflections of a score of men, young men with shaven heads, none of whom I recognize. They stand shoulder to shoulder, blocking me.

What does look familiar is the tattoo on their arms: a scaly snake slithering down the skin, in and out of inked serpentine letters. It is raising its ugly head over each one of their elbows, as if to spit poison around the reddish track marks, caused no doubt by repeated drug injections.

It is the exact same tattoo as the one I saw on Oleg. *Voola.*

This, of course, is no time for polite introductions, but I do my best. I turn around to face the gangsters and, with my loveliest, most beguiling smile, kick the one closest to me as sharply as I can, right in the balls. And as he folds over, grumbling in pain, I push past him and bolt for my Escape.

Chapter 16

Yanking my arms out of their grasp, I skip the three steps down to street level. The gangsters don't immediately follow. They must be confident they can catch up. Why else would they give me a head start?

I stumble over a pile of junk, lose a shoe in the shuffle, kick off the other, and scramble, somehow, across the side street, now hearing them—heavy footfalls, head-splitting shouts—in hot pursuit.

A car stops with a sharp slam of the brakes mere inches from me. "Hey!" yells the driver. Thankfully, it's hard to understand her because she's honking like a crazed goose. I figure she means, "And where the hell d'you think you're going?"

I wave my arms frantically, cry for help—but she just sails on, cursing.

One of the goons comes dangerously close. I feel him breathing down my neck. My energy waning, I try to sprint across the block. Huffing, he claps a hand on my arm. Without thinking twice, I scratch it, drawing blood. He falls back, screaming bloody murder. Jolted, I skip around the corner with a single bound.

There, a second gangster lays his hands on me. He tugs at my blouse, and its back gets ripped apart as I twist away. I hop over some garbage bags heaped on the pavement, grab a broken leg of some discarded piece of furniture, and swing it back at him. It smacks his scalp, hard.

It is then—just as my Escape comes into view—that a third man overtakes me. He grabs me around my waist. No matter how much kicking and screaming I do, he holds firm. Forcing me down, he sets his knee on top of my shoulder blade and clasps my elbows behind my back. In utter agony, I let out a blood-curdling shriek, barely able to recognize this as my voice.

Meanwhile, the others gather all around us, watching the spectacle, panting. Lying flat on the pavement, all I can do is twist my neck and stare helplessly at the front tire of my car. It's been slashed.

What's the point of putting up a fight? From the beginning, this chase was bound to end badly. Up to now, I've sensed no fear—just a flush of adrenaline coursing through my veins, which has so far sustained me, sustained my hope. Now, even that is gone.

My heart is crushed.

Meanwhile, an unidentified gray van comes rolling down the empty street. Suddenly, it hits me. I remember seeing it before. Where was it? Oh yes. *Charmlee Wilderness Park.*

About a week ago, I was hiding there in a ditch, cowering next to Michael. Amidst the debris raining down from the sky and landing all around us, we watched this van as it made a U-turn. The driver smiled broadly at his handiwork. The mangled thing that used to be my boyfriend's Tesla, consumed by flames.

And now, the same van has followed me all the way from Irvine, just like it did Michael. I now recall spotting it in my rearview mirror. Why didn't I pay closer attention to that vehicle? Why didn't I try to lose it?

Climbing down from the van is a big man in camouflage wear with no insignia. He has a wide leather belt and a face shield fixed to his military helmet. Blinded for a second by the flash of the glassy thing, I squint. It takes me a moment to recognize his profile—or rather, to recognize his eyeball. It is marbled with tortuous veins.

Oleg.

He drags me forcibly to my feet. With a hand signal to the other thugs, who are still catching their breath, he mutters, "*Voola*," before throwing me into the back of the van like a sack of potatoes.

Before the van door slides to a close, Oleg hops in next to me. He ties my hands together and blindfolds me. I feel him grabbing my rear.

He grumbles. "Vy so jumpy?"

I recoil, fearing he's again going to force himself on me.

But no, what he does is something that—in his demented mind—must be just as devastating. He gets my cellphone out of my back pocket. No longer do I have a way of calling anyone for help.

Or so he thinks.

"Vat," he says, pulling away. "You got nutting to say?"

Despite the tears, I put on a smile. What Oleg must not know is my little secret: I have a second cellphone on me. It belongs to my boyfriend. I turned it off and have kept it tucked into my bra ever since Michael was hospitalized. No one can guess that it is nestled there, between my boobs. This way, I keep him close to my heart.

On second thought, maybe I should hide it elsewhere. My boobs are not the safest place, given what Oleg is likely to grab.

I used this cellphone only that one time, to watch the virtual reality recording inside the refrigerator truck as it left UCI Medical Center. I recall the bagged corpses that rolled across its corrugated floor. One of them used to be the mastermind of a criminal Russian organization. Vlad. To my surprise, I saw him there, rising to his feet out of an unzipped body bag and jumping off the truck.

Vlad found his way to slip out of the hospital and, at the same time, escape justice. To this day, I find that utterly maddening. I doubt I'll ever have the chance to face him again, let alone exact punishment for what his thug, Oleg, did to me.

A sudden air draft tells me he's just opened the van's sliding door. The driver-side door clicks open. By the thump, he's plopping into the driver seat.

"You ready?" he asks, his tone frighteningly gleeful. "Vee are going to have more fun zen you can take!"

The engine begins to rumble, which covers my cries for help. My body is thrust back into the seat as the van jerks forward. At first, I try to count the twists and turns, try to commit them to memory in precise sequence, so as to map in my mind where I'm being taken.

The idea of communicating my position to the outside world is tempting—if only I could free my hands, get Michael's cellphone out, turn it on, and place a 911 call.

After a while, I lose count of the twists and turns and instead, resign myself to despair. No matter how hard I've tried to release my wrists from the rope that ties them, the only result is nothing to write home about. All I've managed is to chafe my skin to the point of bleeding.

All I can do now, in the blackness wrapped over my eyes, is feel the road. It is bumpy—the rattling shakes me down to my bones—and leads to an unknown destination, unknown fate.

*

The drive seems like forever, which gives me a chance to come out of my fearful silence and instead, strike a conversation with my captor. After all, what do I have to lose?

"Oleg?" I say, struggling to subdue the disgust, the terror I feel in his presence.

My body is thrust forward as he slams on the brakes. "Do not talk to me vile I'm driving."

"Why not?" I ask, teasingly. "You can drive and talk at the same time, no?"

"Vlad varned me about you. He said you vill try to confuse me."

"Vlad isn't here. And he won't know what happens between the two of us. If you don't tell him, I won't, either."

"Oh," says Oleg.

"Besides, you're the one in control. Tied and blindfolded, I am in your hands." I try for a velvety tone. It sounds pretty convincing, if I say so myself. "What danger do I pose to you?"

"All right, zen."

"So, let's forget Vlad."

"Yes," Oleg says. "Forget him."

My first instinct is to ask where he's taking me, but I don't think he's stupid enough to tell me outright. So instead, I go for roundabout chitchat. Anything to diffuse his suspicious attitude and get some answers out of him. "Linda told me a lot about you."

"Oh?" His voice falters into slight hesitation. "Vat she say?"

"She said she thought you're such an important man. A manager at the bank, or something."

He cracks a laugh. "Forget her. Linda vould say anything, do anything to get high. For booze."

"And for drugs, too?"

"Vhere she gets zem who knows. I do not vaste my good stuff on her."

I recall Linda putting on that act of nearly drowning. After I rescued her, she stepped accidentally on a heroin needle that lay discarded on the sand. Serves her right, because she repaid me by stealing my identify.

According to police, that needle carried his DNA. So in all probability, Oleg was there, too, to make sure she did his bidding. Like he says, anything for booze.

While these thoughts flash through my mind, I continue to make small talk. "Linda said you like to go for long walks on the beach. I like it, too."

"Vant us to stop at Pointe Dume? It is close. Vee can go down to beach—"

"Can't," I say. "It's a long way down with no shoes."

"No problem. I give you shoes."

"What?"

"New shoes, belong to Linda. She forget shoes in back of van. Zey good for valking."

What choice do I have but to play along? "Okay," I say, even though I have no idea what awaits me once we get there. "I love that beach."

And he says, "I know."

"Do you? I used to take strolls in the warm sand with my boyfriend."

"I know," he repeats. "I vaited for you. Vith Linda, too."

"You expected me to come? How on earth could you know—"

"Vee vatch you for long time. And vee vatch your boyfriend, too." Oleg chokes a cackle. "Vee know everything vee need to know about both of you."

"Oh, how smart of you!"

"Yes." By the sound of it, he's thumping his chest. "Smart. That's me!"

Flattery works, so I go on to heap more praise on him. "A smooth operation is something I admire. I would even clap my hands for you, Oleg—if only they were free."

"Oh, I do not know about zat." All of a sudden, his voice turns hoarse. "First, say you vant me."

I shudder as he lets out these words. They bring back the scene of my rape. Because I'm deprived of vision, the memory erupts in my mind more vividly than ever. I remember spotting a vague reflection of him in the glass door of my dorm. I remember the pain as he grasped my hair and pulled it, hard.

I remember turning around, my heart pounding at the sound of his sudden hiss. "Say you vant me." And before I knew it, a blow glanced off my chin. In the darkness, I saw a flash of light but couldn't make sense of what was happening, even as the next blow came my way.

And now, with the same inflection, Oleg demands, "Say you vant me."

"How can I say that," I ask, "when I can't even see your face?"

To my surprise, he relents. "I vill soon take off your blindfold."

"Will you untie me, too?"

"Maybe."

"When?"

"Ven vee stop," he says. "Soon."

Chapter 17

Even with eyes strapped, I can tell by the driving maneuvers that the van has pulled into a parking spot. Turns out Oleg is a man of his word, especially when it comes to the prospect of satisfying his own lust. Oh, lucky me! He slides open the door, drags me out of the back seat and—as promised—removes my blindfold.

Vision is not all it's cracked up to be. The sight of him licking his lips with his fat tongue is less than thrilling. His grin bares a gap between his crooked front teeth, through which I could drop a quarter or two. If only my hands were free.

"Now vee go to zeh beach," he mutters, impatiently. "Easy valk, I svear. It is all downhill from here."

I sigh. "You can say that again."

"It is all downhill from here."

No kidding.

At the first step outside the van, my bare feet hit the hard surface. All I can say is, "Ouch."

"Vait." He leans into the open car door, still holding me tight, and grabs a box with brand new walking shoes, which he says Linda forgot in his van. "Put zem on. Hurry."

I fumble with the shoes, not only because my wrists are bound together and fingers are quivering but also because obedience is not exactly my thing. What's the big rush, anyway?

Meanwhile, he takes out a telescopic steel baton and triggers it out. I suppose he just wants to show me his boy toy.

Struggling to hide how nervous it makes me, I just say, "Hey, chill out, will you? Shoestrings aren't the easiest thing to handle with your wrists bound together. If you don't believe me, try it."

He lets out a heavy grunt. Sounds like his heart is about to break. Oh, I can only wish.

"Oleg," I say, "how about, free my hands?"

He lets the baton hang idly by his side, and his eyes start filling with menace. "No vay."

"Oh well." I shrug. "You can't blame me for asking."

Finally, the shoes are on. I straighten, then rub my eyes, trying to keep the rope from itching my nose. Despite the shadows, I recognize this place. Pointe Dume. Near the top of the bluffs, the path passes right along the edge, skirting a sharp drop-off. Seen from here, the ocean should be sparkling in the distance—but on this moonless night, it looks dim.

I remember how lovely this beach looked from this very spot a month ago, how it greeted Michael and me with a beautiful sunset as we clung to each other, kissing.

Clouds were brushing the horizon copper, their fiery edges sketched in reflection across the vast surface of swirling water. An abundance of wildflowers burst over the shoulder of the bluff, painting it mustard yellow. Tickseed flowers shook their toothed-tip petals, their scent sweetening the salty breeze.

The breeze is just as bitter now—but the fragrance has been lost.

His clammy hand paws at my waist, which startles me into the present. It's not where I want to be.

"I vill not hurt you," Oleg tells me, "if you do vat I want."

I know what he wants to hear, what would turn him on—but I'm in no hurry to say it, because of what would inevitably come next.

Drooling, he hisses in my ear, "Say you vant me."

And just as I take a fluttering breath, not even sure what would fly out of my mouth, something unexpected happens. A buzz. It vibrates noisily from his pocket. It's my cellphone, which he's snatched away from me.

Oleg now has three things to juggle: the cellphone, the baton, and me. He does his best. First, he uses his right hand to lean me against the van. With his left, he sticks the baton under his armpit, grabs the cellphone out of his shirt pocket—maybe he mistakes it for his own—then barks, impulsively, "Vat?"

I hear Rita's voice, bright and cheery. "Hi!"

His hold on me is somewhat looser than before, perhaps because he's distracted. The baton keeps slipping from his armpit every time he raises the cellphone to his ear. "Hi," he says, in apparent confusion.

"Who is this?"

"Vat number you call? Zis is mistake."

I don't stick around to hear the rest. Instead, I jerk my elbow sharply out of his hated clasp. And on impulse, I leap off the trail, my body rolling down, bumping over the steep, rocky slope —unfortunately, without the benefit of using my arms for balance.

Oleg is coming for me—his bellow, way up above, is deafening—but at this point, despite getting banged every which way, I feel simply ecstatic. A chill sings around me in the night air. I am free.

For now.

*

It's an hour before sunrise, and Oleg hasn't caught up to me yet. I've counted on him not to leap off the edge after me. Under stress, no one can be as crazy as I am.

Oh, what a blissful silence this is, when his curses and grunts are way behind me, out of hearing range.

I've gotten downhill in one fell swoop, and now I'm limping my way into running. From time to time, I stop just long enough to catch my breath.

Then, at the base of the high rock wall, I use a sharp edge of one of the boulders to rub, to abrade the rope tying my hands till its fibers get frayed, till at long last it is undone, and my wounded hands are released from bondage.

By now, the tide has receded, but the water is too rough to walk through. I take off the shoes, tie their shoestrings together and hang the knotted pair on my shoulder, before scrambling barefoot behind the boulders. Even as I climb, I'm sprayed by the waves sloshing constantly in and out of little pools and, from time to time, surging over the rocks with a frothy splash. I clamber over stone surfaces and, at last, find the rugged path leading to Pirates Cove.

Here, the long patch of sand—nestled amidst vertical stone surfaces—looks so soft, so inviting, calling me to sink my toes in. For fear of leaving traces, I resist the temptation. Instead, I cower behind one of the rocks strewn around the periphery, pull Michael's cellphone out of my bra, and turn it on.

How it managed to stay tucked in there, despite everything I went throughout this horrific night, is nothing short of a miracle. There's something to be said about big boobs.

Last time I called Rita, it was from my own cellphone—not from Michael's. I have her number memorized. I punch it, wondering if she'll pick up the call.

Rita doesn't answer the first time, nor the second. I imagine her wiping sleep from her eyes, then staring at the caller ID, unable to recognize it. She must be wondering who might be calling at this godforsaken hour.

Third time is the charm.

"Oh, it's you." She yawns. "I called you earlier and someone else answered. I could barely understand a word he said."

"That's Oleg."

"Oleg who?"

"I'll tell you all about him, but not now—"

"Oh Ash, I was so worried!"

"So was I, Rita—"

She goes into gushing, "I thought I'll never hear your voice again!"

I have to admit, "I had my doubts, too."

"Is he next to you?"

"No, but—"

"Good. Glad you got away. Where the heck are you now?"

"Pirate's Cove."

"Ah! I suppose this isn't a romantic getaway?"

"*Getaway* it is, *romantic*—not so much."

Sigh. Usually, Rita is quick-witted—but not this time. She seems not to have figured my urgent need to get the hell out of this little haven.

"On a different note, I got the pics you sent," she prattles in her perky manner, which makes it hard for me to cut in. "These fraud complaints, written by several insurance beneficiaries, are quite telling. What a scoop! Thank you, thank you! By now, I've checked around, done some research about that dermatology clinic, and—"

"Will you shut up and listen?" I butt in. "I'm in a bind here. Need help. Now."

"Oh?" says Rita. "Why, what's happening?"

"I'm being chased by a Russian gorilla."

"This Oleg guy?"

"Yes."

"Oh no!"

"He tied my hands together."

"Oh no, no!"

"And Rita, he came at me with a baton."

"Oh my God!"

"And now, he's in hot pursuit—"

"Oh, how horrible!"

"But here's the good news."

"What?" She snaps. "What can possibly be good news, when you're on the run?"

I wink. "Got me a new pair of shoes."

"You kidding, right?"

"Why, you think it's funny?"

"Not really, Ash. When did you find time to go shopping?"

"Don't even ask."

She doesn't. Instead, she puts me quickly on hold. I wait till she calls 911 on my behalf, then till she's done talking with her police friend, so he can help speed things up to extricate me out of this place, pronto.

Meanwhile, I call UCI Medical Center and ask for an update on the status of Michael Morse. The secretary checks her records and tells me the patient has already been released, early this morning. Last she heard, he's been trying to call me, repeatedly.

Rita's back on line. She tells me that the police have been contacted and a rescue mission is in the works.

"Can't wait," I say.

And she says, "Me neither."

"I mean, really. If Oleg shows up, which can happen any moment now, I'll have to slip away somehow, God knows where."

"Hang on, Ash. The cops will be there, soon."

"Thank you." An agitated sigh escapes my throat. "Rita, can you do me one more favor?"

"Anything."

"Can you contact my boyfriend?"

"Why can't you call him?"

"Because, Rita, he doesn't have his cellphone. I have it."

"And what about email?"

"I have no access to my email. For the life of me I can't remember the damn password. So will you do it for me?" I give her his email.

"Sure. Consider it done."

"I'm told he was trying to call me from the hospital. Tell him I can only be reached through *his* number—not mine."

"I will. No problem."

"Michael will know what to do. He'll track his own cellphone to know where I am."

"Got it. Talk soon."

Fifteen minutes later, I call her again, my anxiety reaching a new high. I've been perking my ears, straining to hear the engine of a police watercraft coming for me any moment now—but so far, crickets.

"Where are the cops when you need them? Or the Coast Guard? Or anyone?"

"They're on the way."

"Are they?"

"Relax, Ash. Just sit tight—"

"Easy for you to say." Any moment now, Oleg may find his way into the Cove. I hope the cops can make it here before he does. "How will they get here? By boat?"

"No. There are too many rocks in the water, so maneuvering around them will slow down the rescue and put the boat in danger."

"Oh. Will they climb down from the ledge with ropes?"

"No," she says. "That's just as risky. I can't imagine how they'll climb back up carrying you."

"If not by sea, not by land, then what?" I scratch my head, a bit bewildered. "How will they get me out of here?"

"By air," says Rita. "Stay tuned."

Chapter 18

My latest discovery: I'm black and blue all over. My blouse is ripped at the back, and my jeans—more frayed than is fashionably acceptable. The only thing about me that is still intact is my manicure—until I begin to bite my nails.

To keep from going crazy while waiting in Pirate's Cove to be rescued, I squat on a patch of sand and build a sandcastle. Then, I lie next to it, the curve of my hip rising above the dip of my waist like a knocked over hourglass. I count time. Heartbeats. Grains of sand. They flow between my fingers, then spread out in the breeze. The feel is soothing to me. It harkens back to happier times.

The last word from Rita: a rescue operation has been dispatched, to be executed by the Los Angeles County Sheriff's Helicopter. Also, a Nixle alert has just been issued. It is texted to tens of thousands of subscribers—this cellphone included—advising them that a helicopter is in the city, responding to a distress call at Pirate's Cove.

I tuck the cellphone into my bra, which is the least probable place for that purpose, just in case I get caught by Oleg before my saviors arrive. And just as I hide it, a ping makes my heart skip a beat. The call is coming from an unfamiliar number.

"Hello?" I say.

"Hi, sweetheart."

"Oh! It's you, Michael!"

He sounds downright worried. "Hope you're not in trouble?"

"Me? Ha! Never." My attempt at humor fails miserably, because of the quiver that takes over my voice. I try again. "I'm safe and sound, babe, but you beware. Trouble is my middle name."

"I don't mind," he counters. "It's your *last* name I'm hoping to change."

"But Michael," I say, digging my toes in the sand, "I like the ring of Winters."

"Imagine the ring of Morse."

"I'll have to say it over and again, because it sounds strange to my ears."

He chuckles. "Well, get used to it, because I'm in love with you, the future Mrs. Morse."

"Is that your way of asking for my hand?"

"No, sweetheart. When I propose, you'll have absolutely no doubt about my intentions."

With my finger, I draw a door on my sandcastle and underline it to indicate a threshold.

"Ash, you still there?"

"Not going anywhere, yet."

"Seriously now," he says. "I hear there's an alert. Hope it's not about you?"

I let out a sigh.

"Ash?"

"Yes," I admit. "It's me alright."

"I knew it!"

I blink back tears. "Wish you were here."

"One way or another," he says, "I will be. I'll come to your help. That's a promise."

"Where are you now? I thought you were heading home from the hospital—"

"Not anymore. I'm on my way to you."

"Really?" I take a deep breath, hoping for a quick relief. "How? Last I saw, your Tesla went out in flames—"

"Got me an Uber. Didn't you notice the number I'm calling from? It belongs to my driver."

"When will you be here?"

"An hour."

"By the time you arrive, I'll be lifted out of here."

"Keep my cellphone on you at all times," he says. "Its GPS tells me where you are."

"Okay, Michael. Love you."

"Love you too, sweetheart. And oh, whatever you do, don't hang up."

A repeat of the Nixle alert flashes across the screen. I wonder: is Michael the only one who's leapt to the conclusion that this rescue is meant for me?

Oleg is not known for his wits. Chances are, he doesn't even subscribe to Nixle alerts—or else he would be heading this way right now, to offer the one specialty he's proud of: bringing a world of hurt on me.

Being a simple-minded thug, Oleg can't be a high-ranking member of the gang. Someone else is organizing it, someone smart enough to plan a large-scale insurance fraud and to thwart any attempts to expose it.

I glance at the Nixle alert. Whoever that person is, I hope he's not paying attention.

*

Staying in the shade, I hang my eyes on the sky. At the end of an impossibly stretched-out forever, a faint silhouette clears out of the cloud that hangs over the bluffs. I listen anxiously for the incoming sound. Chuffing as it comes, the helicopter whirls over, blades rotating, slapping the air with a swish-swash-swish-swash sound.

Despite my aching limbs, I hop to my feet and come out from behind the rocks. Sunlight has just begun to wash over the beachfront. The closer the helicopter comes—the larger its shadow, fluttering fluidly towards me across the ground.

Squinting, I flail my arms to make sure the pilot spots me. Blindingly sharp rays of sun are bouncing off its long metal skids.

There is barely any vegetation here to help the crew determine the velocity of the wind and its direction. Instead, smoke is used to guide the flight maneuvers. Something is thrust out of the helicopter, letting out a wisp of fume that spirals thinly in the air as the thing flies, as it pins itself into the sand at the other side of my castle.

After a few adjustments back and forth, the helicopter settles overhead into position. The rotor whips the air into a frenzy. Sand lifts into a swirl around me. The entire view is seen through a trembling sheet of vapor. It separates into layers, some of them transparent, some opaque. I am awash in salty droplets that fly at me. Mist is billowing all around.

I draw in a deep breath, taking it all in. My chest swells, my lungs expand. Still, I feel dizzy, this time with an intoxicating sense of relief. I'm going to make it, going to be airlifted to safety!

A crew member, secured in a hoisting vest fitted over a full body suit, is lowered via a cable to the surface. Wearing a helmet visor in addition to safety goggles, flight protective gloves, and a respirator mask, he looks like an alien. I suppose a rescue operation in the middle of a raging pandemic is nothing to sneeze at.

His voice filters through the mask. "You injured?"

"Nothing serious," I say. "Just banged a bit here and there."

With proficient moves, he unfolds the rescue harness and starts packaging me into it, adding layers of PPE: a gown, gloves, and double sheets to provide as much barrier as possible between us, just as a precaution, in case I have some respiratory problem.

"Put the harness on. Hands go here, like you're putting on a coat," he instructs. "Good. Your outcome depends on a timely transport to medical care."

"A timely transport is just… Just what I want." My voice becomes muffled mid-sentence, as he fits a respirator mask on my face. My excitement subdued, I turn silent.

A cable is lowered from the helicopter. The rescuer snaps its hook securely into my harness. "All set," he says, and before I know it, both of us are dangling together off the ground.

Out of the corner of my eye, I spot someone running across the beach, waving his hands, thrashing about frantically.

"Vait!" Oleg cries. "Vait for me!"

The thug goes on yelling. He curses me, curses himself for being too late for the party. As I rise, the sound of the rotor overhead is becoming strong enough to drown out his voice. After a while, Oleg becomes a distant dot.

He can't get me. I'm safe.

*

My earlier dizziness is nothing compared to how disoriented I feel, now that I've lost touch with the ground. The entire view is tilting precariously, falling farther and farther down below us. The higher we ascend, the greater my confusion.

If not for this harness pressing against my ribs, I should feel as free as a bird. But that's not how I find myself, even though I try. I spread out my arms and flap them about as if they were wings. All the while, some little voice in my head is screaming. I cup my ears—to no avail. I can still hear it cry.

Danger.

So far, we've been hoisted to the level of the landing gear. My rescuer gives a nod to someone just above us. The hoist operator. Wearing a full body suit, he stands just outside the helicopter, his boots on the metal skid, ready to help us into the cabin. Boy, do I envy him! He must feel on top of the world.

A moment later, his hand curls around my waist, pulling me in.

I'm lying on the floor, watchful of the surroundings. Besides the pilot, who keeps his eyes steadily on the controls with his back to me, there's one more crew member. He's masked, just like my rescuer. I suppose that's per standard isolation protocols. Except for his icy-blue eyes, I can spot no facial features. He must be a medic. Or so I figure, at first.

Strangely, this man is in no hurry to check my injuries or even release the harness, in which I'm confined. Instead, he extends his hand and grabs mine. I respond to his handshake with an agonized smile. It can crack an egg.

Outside, the hoist operator begins pushing my rescuer into the cabin. It is then that the incredible happens.

The so-called medic releases my hand and turns to them. "Stand back," he says. "We have a problem." His voice sounds terribly familiar, and so does his British accent.

"What?" asks the hoist operator, leaning into the opening from outside the craft.

And my rescuer, his hands reaching over the threshold, brushing across the floor as if to feel for a grip, echoes after him, "What?"

"I said, stand back," stresses the so-called medic. "That goes for both of you."

I listen for any telltale slips in his British pronunciation, in vain. It's too perfect. Language is history. It reveals the past. His skill at concealing his is unmatched. But now I know who he is and what he's capable of.

With a sleek jerk, he unhooks the hoist operator from whatever it is that has so far secured him to the craft.

"Stop!" cries the operator, clearly in shock. For the first time, he seems shaky on his feet, struggling to keep his balance out there. "What the hell are you doing? What's your problem?"

"It's simple, really," says the man. His tone is polite, but cold. "I have no more need for you."

He steps onto the knuckles of my rescuer, and his eyes fill with pleasure at the sound of cracking. And with a whack, he sends his knee into the hoist operator's groin. "SasviDAniya," the man mutters, this time in Russian. By his tone of finality, I know what it means. Good bye.

Folding in pain, the victim slips off the skid, his arms thrashing about. A shriek sears the air, then wanes to eerie silence, as he is sucked away.

Meanwhile, the bloodied fingers of my rescuer are slow to peel off the threshold—until at last he gives up his grasp. A thump comes from below. By the sudden shaking of the aircraft, I figure his body must have been jolted against the landing gear. Perhaps he's caught hold of it, somehow, under the belly of the helicopter. I imagine him hanging there, clinging for dear life.

Not for long.

Meeting a similar fate would be nothing to write home about. So, I wiggle quickly out of the harness and roll to my knees, ready to protect myself.

The man comes over to me with a swift step. To my astonishment, he offers a hand to help me to my feet, as if he were a perfect gentleman, as if the killing of two crew members never happened, it was but a strange mirage or a distant memory with no bearing on the present. "Hello, Ashley Winters. I haven't forgotten you."

I recoil. "Hello, Vlad Komarov. I wish you would."

He strips off his mask, then steps back, allowing me the space to rise on my own. "It's been a while. You look as stunning as ever."

"You look well, for a change. Got tired of playing dead?"

"Playing dead is one hell of a way to avoid paying a price for what I did. As you must know, being in a coma is no fun, especially if you have to fake it."

"Tell me about it."

"I'd like to believe you've missed my company. I've certainly missed yours."

Vlad reaches over, perhaps to test my reaction. He touches my arm lightly, in the tender manner of lovers, almost.

I swing it back at him.

He sighs. "I forgot how difficult you can be."

Turning sideway, he gives a quick signal to the pilot, and the helicopter changes course.

Bloody fingerprints glisten over the edge, an indelible reminder of what I've just witnessed. I gaze at the cable that has hoisted me, now snaking uncontrollably across the floor and rattling to a rest at his feet.

Vlad must have received word of my location and managed to intercept the rescue with an operation of his own. I figure he used some connections to replace the pilot and board the craft, posing as a medic. All that, at a moment's notice. Against my will, I'm impressed with his efficiency as well as his daring.

"Vlad?" I search his eyes, finding emptiness. "You've gone to a lot of trouble to arrange this meeting between us, such as it is—"

"Let's call it a date, shall we? You may have your reasons for it, I have mine." He bares his teeth, the corners of his mouth curling in a sharp way into something that can't be called a smile. "Either way, we both know it is long overdue."

"What is it that you want from me?"

"You will find out soon enough."

Chapter 19

Vlad tells the pilot to head to The Ronald Reagan UCLA Medical Center, because the flight may be tracked on radar by police. In his words, "We better give the bastards exactly what they expect." But on the way there, he points at a particular flat rooftop somewhere on the outskirts of Los Angeles and demands a landing, for just a moment. His purpose is surprising: to bring aboard another woman.

She climbs in, averting her eyes from me, bestowing a smile on Vlad. Then, at takeoff, a gust of wind makes the wig tilt over her head, nearly knocking it over. It is at that second that I know for sure: this is Linda Leigh.

"Ah!" Vlad claps his hands in mock applause. "My favorite actress."

I don't quite understand her role in his mission—or my own role for that matter. The first clue happens when he tells me to pull down my jeans.

"What?" I cry. "No way!"

He cracks a laugh. "You think you have much choice in this matter?"

"You think I've lost my mind?"

Meanwhile, Linda starts undressing in plain sight. She acts as if this were her private dressing room—only more upscale, with a spectacular view of Los Angeles dropping away and clouds wafting by.

"Don't be stubborn," Vlad tells me. "I'm going to turn my back and not even take a peek, if it's me you're worried about."

And, playing the perfect gentleman, he does.

By now, Linda is down to her panties and goosebumps, which doesn't prevent her from a show of hostility towards me. She takes her pistol out of her purse and, with a shaky hand, puts it to my temple. "Do as you're told. And hurry. I'm cold."

I'm getting tired of threats, so I snap at her. "Shoot me now, see if I care! Why should I be the one to freeze?"

Linda lowers her pistol and shoves her bunched-up skirt and sweater into my hands. "Here. Put them on. And give me your blouse. Your bra, too."

I decide to relent, not so much because I'm afraid, but because her lips are turning blue. "Mind if I turn my back?"

She shrugs. "As long as you do it in a snap, I don't mind if you spin around like a top."

Facing away from both of them as I strip is not a matter of modesty. I've never been shy about my boobs. But Michael's cellphone, tucked in-between them, is nobody's business but mine. I pray that my love is still listening at the other end and mapping out my position, somewhere between heaven and earth. He's my last lifeline.

Linda taps her foot impatiently. Her teeth are chattering. "Hey, I'm waiting."

Keeping a watchful eye on Vlad over my shoulder, I drop my jeans to the floor and, with a flair, kick them backwards to her. If he's hoped to see me in my panties, I have a surprise for him.

They're covered by my spandex leggings. There's something to be said about dressing in layers.

I unfold her clothes, turning my nose away from the body odor infused in them, and pull up her black skirt. As fashion goes, it is just my style, featuring silvery snap buttons down the front and a sexy cut, designed to show off the hips. I fasten it around my waist, then shimmy out of my blouse. I leave on my tie-dyed undershirt because she didn't ask for it.

Under it, I hold on to the cellphone with one hand. With the other, I remove my bra—letting it all shake loose—and toss it over to Linda, although heaven knows she has no real need for it. All the while, my mind is racing. I'm desperate to find a new hiding place for the cellphone.

In a bind, the black sweater offers a solution. While Vlad is looking the other way, I shove the cellphone halfway down its sleeve. To secure the thing in place, I double-tie the left sleeve with the right, then casually fling the sweater over my shoulders as if this is nothing more than a fashion statement.

"My sweater is going to get out of shape that way," she complains. "Why aren't you putting it on?"

"Because," I say, "I'm too hot."

I press the knot, with the cellphone in it, over my heart. My nipples are dancing freely against my undershirt, which makes Linda flash an envious look. By now, she has packed herself into my jeans, fixed the wig to sit properly on her head, and true to form, dons not only my bra and blouse but also my persona, apparently in preparation for her role after the landing.

I notice she's dropped the pistol into her purse and is no longer posing an immediate threat to me. So I slide over the bench next to her. "Why are you doing this?" I whisper.

Her breath smells of Vodka. "Huh? What?"

"Didn't you tell me, last time we met, that stealing my identity was a bad deal for you? Didn't you say you were falsely led to believe there were tens of thousands of dollars in my bank account? Now, don't be a fool—"

"I may have made a mistake back then, but a fool I'm not," she insists.

"You also stated that playing me is no fun—"

"Trying to cope with my life is no fun either. No job. No booze. No way to afford my chemo treatments." Linda casts a timid look at Vlad, who is still facing away, pretending not to hear us. "To get what I need, I have to be creative."

"You mean, you have to steal?" I try reaching out to her one more time. If I can convince her to come to her senses, maybe we can work together. Maybe we can overpower him. "Didn't you admit to me that the crime cost you dearly? That you were being blackmailed for it?"

Her eyes are bloodshot. "I'm only too happy to be blackmailed into doing one more job. It gets me to the next day."

"It's more than a job," Vlad says, out of the blue. "Given an impeccable performance, it can turn into the role of a lifetime."

A clownish smile plays in the corners of her mouth. It seems to be born out of despair. "Really?"

"Really," says Vlad. "I knew you're the one to pull it off, when I saw you in *Midsummer Night's Dream*. What a star you are!"

"Oh." Her face reddens. "Thank you."

"You know my favorite part?"

"No, Vlad. What is it?"

"It's the line, 'Die, die, die, die, die,' from the Pyramus and Thisbe play-within-a-play."

"Oh." She lowers her eyes, clearly in disappointment, and her blush fades away. "That's not my line."

"No," he says. "It isn't."

Linda collects herself, somehow, into sounding agreeable. "Dying onstage can look like a ridiculously prolonged agony."

"Yes. More so than in real life."

She nods.

A second later, he reflects on it again. "In real life, I like things cut and dry."

✳

While they busy themselves with this lofty literary exchange, the helicopter is nearing the helipad on the roof of the north side of UCLA Medical Center. My heart starts hammering. I slide away from Linda and wonder out loud if the medical teams would arrive at once. If they do, perhaps I can signal for help.

Breaking his silence, the pilot responds. "No," he says. "They're waiting inside until the helicopter lands, until it throttles down."

Vlad snaps at him. "You, shut up! Keep your eyes on the controls and your yap closed. And you," he says to Linda, his voice turning frosty all of a sudden. "Who said you can bring a weapon onboard? Don't you know that's forbidden?"

"Sorry," she says, meekly now.

He sticks out an open palm. "Give it to me."

Not daring to disobey, she does.

Vlad grabs her pistol, opens a plastic box marked with a red cross and places the thing under a bunch of medical supplies. Then he checks his watch, nods in apparent satisfaction, even chuckles. Apparently, everything is going according to plan. Seems like it's time for his next step.

With a sudden pull, he twists her arm behind her back till she screams, "Why?"

"I hate having to explain things to you, Linda darling. I won't stand for mistakes."

"But—but—I didn't know—I said I was sorry—"

"In my organization," he says proudly, while forcing her to her knees, "things run with cutthroat efficiency."

She starts sobbing.

"I'll tell you a little story," he hisses, leaning into her ear. "Do we have enough time? Yes, I think we do. You listening?"

She nods.

Vlad takes out a white handkerchief, wipes her wet face. Her neck, too. "Born in Moscow, brought up in London, I soaked in the culture of both East and West. From early childhood, I had great gifts. Admired by my peers, I learned languages with great ease, excelled in every subject, and was considered quick-witted. Then, in a moment of rage, I killed a man. It was at that point that I found I possessed another gift: I could commit murder without remorse."

While Vlad is telling her about his past, I entertain some hope —slim as it may seem—that this is all talk, that he doesn't really mean her any harm. Until, in a flash, he produces a knife, who knows from where, and slashes her neck.

"Here's a Russian proverb my darling Mamushka used to tell me." He takes his sweet time wiping the blood from his knife, then smiles at her tortured expression. "*Don't blame the mirror for your ugly face.*"

As blood spurts out of her lacerated carotid artery—as the life drains out of her—Vlad rolls the dying woman onto a stretcher and wraps her in plastic sheets. He checks her pulse, waits a moment, checks it again. Then, he selects one of the bandages in his box and wraps it slowly, meticulously around her wounded neck, with the well-practiced motions of a medic. But she is beyond saving. Too little, too late.

Finally, we land. When the medics arrive, Vlad tells them, "The patient's name? Ashley Winters. We lifted her out of Pirate's Cove. She's in critical condition."

To that he adds that another distress call has just come in. With an agile step, he hops back into the helicopter and signals the pilot to take off at once. A moment later, we're in the air.

After that, I find myself in shock.

It takes me a long while to still my racing heart, to compose myself. Earlier, I saw Vlad push two crew members—my rescuer and the hoist operator—out of the helicopter, but they met their death out of my sight. I could only imagine their mangled bodies coming to a rest. Not so Linda. Her last convulsions, right in front of me, have stirred me to the core.

Finally, I bring myself to talk. "Why did she have to die?"

"Because." He gives a slight shrug. "She's dispensable. Look, mine is a complicated business. I simply can't rely on a drunk. Her heroin addiction is a liability I can't afford."

"Then why did you bring her aboard?"

Instead of an answer, he says, "Now, think of it: her death has set you free."

Utterly spent, I barely raise an eyebrow. "Free?"

"No one knows you're alive. So if you're smart, you can leave your old life behind. You can serve me." At this point, his tone is fully magnanimous. "A life of crime can be illustrious. Not a dull moment. And mark my word: you'll be handsomely rewarded."

"And if I don't?"

"You die."

"I thought Linda is your favorite actress."

"Yes. That she was," Vlad says, looking me straight in the eye. "Until now."

Chapter 20

As the helicopter takes off from the roof of UCLA Medical Center, Vlad tells the pilot to head to a parking lot at a remote beach and let us out. On the way there, he establishes radio communication with his gang.

"Get the van and meet us, you know where," Vlad says. "And make sure you are not being followed."

An all-too-familiar voice asks, "Vere you need me take you?"

"Headquarters."

"Vill do."

"And Oleg? I know all about your little shenanigans. I suggest you just stop—or else."

"Shenanigans? Me? Vat you mean?"

"Do not, under any circumstances, get your dirty paws on my companion." Vlad shoots a look at me out of the corner of his eye. "She's mine."

Oleg clears his throat, and hesitation creeps in. "Vat's her name?"

"As far as you are concerned, she has none."

*

Having gone through a rough helicopter ride, then a sickeningly tortuous drive in Vlad's van through the streets of Los Angeles, I long for a dull moment. No such luck. Now, I am being escorted along Main street. Well, *Escorted* is not exactly the right word. *Rushed* is more like it.

I keep my eyes down, skipping the cracks in the pavement, watching my shadow being trampled upon. I cast a look sideways at the slightly warped glass of one storefront after another, all showing my reflection, flanked by other reflections, reflections of broad-shouldered gang members—two scores of them, give or take—with tattooed arms.

Vlad marches in the lead. With a crumpled handkerchief, he wipes beads of sweat off the back of his neck. The flesh around his ears seems to squeeze them out of his head by force. His earlobes droop like minced meat out of a grinder.

I glance over my shoulder, hoping to find some way to escape. There isn't any. Oleg follows closely behind me, his sausage fingers hanging idly by his sides, his fat tongue licking his bottom lip.

I'm trapped.

This street seemed eerie last night. In the light of day, it feels even freakier. The first store sign—Cap & Hat Imports—had its first letter dangling on a nail. Now, its *Imports* is missing altogether. Next door, the *Store Closing Sale* sign has been peeled, in jagged scraps, off the glass of The Dish Factory.

The junk that was piled outside the boarded-up storefront has been cleared away. Only a few empty plastic bags remain, some clinging tightly to the pavement, others—lifted by a sudden gust and tossed around. Seen against the afternoon light, their flimsy material is translucent, and the shapes they assume—ghastly.

The plastic bags rustle past us and again, the view is clear. There, across a side street and up three stairs, is where we're headed. The dermatology clinic that never existed.

Vlad cracks his knuckles, then sticks a key in the lock, turns it with a slight squeak, and flings the door wide open. With a most gallant gesture, which I take as an exercise in mockery, he says, "Ladies first," and lets me in. Then, he tells Oleg to stay outside, be on the lookout. Once the rest of the men get in, Vlad latches the door and pockets the key.

"Everyone must make adjustments nowadays because of the pandemic, me included," Vlad says, as if to apologize for the less-than-glamorous interior.

It's empty, except for a long, bare metal table and a few carton boxes stacked under it on a layer of dust. In the corner of the space, one box is open. It is filled with party supplies that no one has a need for these days, because no large gatherings are allowed. A lone helium balloon still hovers just over the floor, a reminder of happier times. No wonder the party store that used to rent this space went out of business.

Small talk never hurt anyone. So, just to keep Vlad chatting, "True," I say. "We must all adapt."

"Especially true," Vlad says, "for criminal enterprises such as mine. Unfortunately, in recent months there's been a severe reduction in crime, including burglaries, because damn it, people stay put in their homes. So, I ask you, what's a thief to do?"

I shrug. "Set his eyes on a different target?"

"Ha! You and I think alike." A smile creeps from one ear to the other. It pushes up his scarred cheeks and stops short of his eyes.

I make an effort not to raise an eyebrow. "We do?"

"I've been told that crawling into my mind is not easy," Vlad says, with unmistakable pride. "For some, it may be downright scary. But then, you—you seem to understand me."

"I try."

"I have fond memories of you visiting me at UCI Medical Center. I never turned to look at you back then—how could I? That would have blown my cover. Still, I found your company quite entertaining. I sensed that having a strikingly beautiful woman at my bedside became the envy of patients and doctors alike. It helped alleviate the gloom of that place, the incessant boredom."

I can't help but cry, "Just as I suspected! Somehow, you managed to fake being in a coma."

"Indeed, that gave me some pleasure. Ha! Those idiots! They thought I was dying."

"Which, quite conveniently, kept you out of paying the price for your crimes."

Vlad chokes a laugh. "Paying a price for anything is not something I do."

I reflect on that, while giving him my most beguiling smile. "May I ask, how did you manage to pull it off?"

"You may," Vlad says, beaming magnanimously. "I had an accomplice. You'll meet her soon enough. She managed the impossible: fooling the doctors by doctoring the readouts of the instruments to which I was connected."

"Really," I say, making sure to add a flattering note. "What a brilliant mind she has!"

Vlad drags a hand down his face and the smile is gone. "Despite playing a vegetable—which as you may know, is quite a stretch—my stay at the hospital was not all fun and games. I realized, of course, that it would cost me dearly."

"In what way?"

"Well, my men lost faith. Some of them joined rival gangs. Others dispersed. My enterprise collapsed altogether."

"Must have been tough for you."

"Tough it was. Besides, I was in danger of getting sick for real. After all, the virus mowed down every patient around me. A few of the nurses, too. Corpses were taken off life support and driven out."

"So, you decided to join them on their last journey."

Startled, Vlad gives me a look. "How did you know?"

"Just a wild guess."

"Not many people can venture into my devious mind. But somehow, you do." He chuckles maliciously. "And you're right. As a corpse, I could finally bolt from the hospital without the police coming to sniff me out."

"Amazing," I say. "The life of a corpse can be full of adventure."

"All I had to do was play dead and trust my accomplice to deliver me back into the land of the living."

"How did she manage that?"

"She forged a signature on my death certificate, hung a tag on my toe, and zipped me up in my snug body bag so everyone mistook me for a stiff. The medical staff loaded me onto the metal floor of a refrigerator truck. Soon after, the engine started. Ah, it was music to my ears! After a short rock and roll among the other body bags, I darted out."

He doesn't mention the brief encounter he had with my boyfriend aboard that truck, and neither do I. But this I know: after Michael followed him, his Tesla went up in smoke.

In Vlad's circles, that counts as a subtle warning.

I bat my eyelashes at him and lick my lips, ever so seductively. "And then?"

"Then, I found myself eager to restart my organization somewhere, somehow. In a pinch, I set my eyes on car theft."

"Car theft? Why?"

"Because, given the Shelter-in-Place restrictions, owners leave their vehicles on the street for days on end and check on them rather infrequently, if at all. With less foot traffic in the street and fewer people to take note, the van was an easy steal."

"And what about this office space? How did you manage to get it?"

"Breaking and entering, what else?"

"Of course, Vlad. What was I thinking?"

"The owner of the building hasn't been here for weeks, as the commercial rental business is on the brink of collapse."

"Nice place," I say. "And the price is right."

His jaw clenches. "No, nice it isn't. This used to be a party store, so my men had to clear away the mess, boxes and boxes of party supplies." He kicks a box full of confetti out of the way. "This place will have to do, for now."

"Oh? You have plans?"

"Soon—if things go my way—we'll be able to splurge on a new office tower and a fleet of cars. Big money is about to roll in. Big, I tell you! Mark my word," he stresses, raising his voice as if to impress not only me but also the others. "Given this fraud scheme, there will be no more need for petty crime!"

While they hoot, Vlad leans, rather intimately, closer to me. His breath is hot on my ear. "That's why I brought you here. I need you to do some work for me."

In the past, his fingerprints were found in several muddy projects, from the shutoff of the electrical grid in the entire state of California, to kidnapping, to child trafficking. Wary of his intentions, I ask, "What kind of work?"

"This is not about sex or drugs or anything violent, so don't you worry." He lets out a heavy grunt. "Insurance fraud is a white-collar crime. It is boring. Benign, too. For the most part, no one gets hurt."

"No one," I daresay, "except for people whose identities get stolen, some of whom reach the point of committing suicide."

He doesn't even blink. "Collateral damage."

"Oh? I thought you said, 'No one gets hurt.'"

"I said, 'For the most part.'" His eyes bore into mine. "Beware. I can see where you're going with all this."

I struggle not to be sucked into the emptiness of his gaze. "Really? Can you?"

"You are thinking about that bitch, what's her name, Linda Leigh."

In surprise, I have to admit, "I am."

"Well, don't. She got what was coming to her." Vlad turns his back on his men. They are clustering at the opposite side of the space, drinking beer, spitting. "From time to time, I have to slit a throat, if only to keep the others in line."

All the while, I try to ignore the new fear that starts gnawing in my stomach. The way Vlad whispers his secrets in my ear suggests that somehow, I've earned his trust. That may seem reassuring—but in truth, it bodes ill for me. He may open doors like a gentleman, but closes them like a brute.

Will Vlad ever let me out of his sight? His attraction to me ends at the edge of this space, and that's where his vengeance begins.

"You haven't answered my question," I say. "What kind of work do you need from me?"

"It involves some clerical machinations. As you can see," he says, hinting at the others, "I'm short of capable staff."

Meanwhile, as if to prove his point, his mysterious accomplice—a heavy set woman in her late sixties—comes in through an inner door I haven't noticed up to now. There is no small talk between her and Vlad, not as much as a nod. In the absence of any exchange, any note of recognition, the air around them seems to tighten.

The men at the opposite side of the space freeze. "Mrs. Komarov is here," one of them whispers, and they all stiffen.

And for the first time since I met him, Vlad draws himself up into tense attention.

Mrs. Komarov is heavy-footed. She works her way in, her manner rigid, her face—severe. "Where's Linda?"

"Indisposed," Vlad says, and everyone around me chuckles nervously, as if they get it, they know what kind of fate she must have met.

Over the rim of her glasses, slipped halfway down her nose, Mrs. Komarov hangs her eyes on him. They're icy blue, just like his. "I'm disappointed in you," she tells him. "There is a right time and a wrong time for everything."

"A lecture from you is the last thing I need—"

"Even so, son," she croaks, "you are going to get it."

"Oh, hush," he hisses. "Everyone is listening—"

"So? You think I care?"

"Please, Mamushka. Not now—"

"In case you haven't noticed, you are in trouble."

Her manner of pronunciation is different than his. It has more than a hint of Russian, overpowering her attempt at a posh accent. No matter how long her stay in England might have been, she has not managed to parrot her British neighbors.

"In trouble?" Vlad echoes, adding an incredulous tone. "And I thought I'm on top of the world."

Mrs. Komarov stamps her foot. "My suggestion is, take a second look."

"I have risen from the dead. No one can take me down!"

"You are on top of a mountain of lies. It is about to collapse under you."

His voice falters. "Have you looked into the paperwork?"

"It is pure crap!" she yells. "I cannot make sense of any of the medical codes you used. Worst of all, an official inquiry—coordinated among several insurance companies—has been started."

"I'm ready for it."

"Are you?"

Vlad takes a deep breath, and his chest swells with pride. "It's from you that I learned the Russian proverb, '*If you're afraid of wolves, don't go to the woods.*'"

Mrs. Komarov pokes him with a sharp nail. "The wolves are coming here. They are coming for you, because the air is heavy with the smell of blood."

He shrinks like a punctured balloon, air rushing out of his mouth. "Ah, nonsense!"

"What exactly have you done to Linda?"

"Nothing worth talking about."

Mrs. Komarov clicks her tongue. "While alive, that woman posed a risk for our business, and the risk is even greater now that she's gone."

He lowers his eyes, stares at his hands. "Talking about her is a waste of time—"

"You want us to be efficient? Fine! Here's something that I find most pressing. These insurance companies, they are looking into the validity of our claims and, in some cases, asking for detailed clarifications."

"So?" He shrugs. "Who cares?"

"I do!" She puts her foot down, which startles him. "We need to provide answers that will, in some manner, satisfy their curiosity or send them chasing some other culprit. We must do so very soon—or else they will become even more suspicious."

Vlad brushes her aside. "What the hell does that matter? Some of these claims will succeed. They will sail through the system, no questions asked. For these, we'll get paid. Big money. Then, we will disappear. We will reinvent ourselves, embark on a new enterprise or something."

"Oh, not again."

"Enough! Just stop this pointless yapping. I am growing tired of it."

The old woman is relentless. She won't be easily silenced. "What I am worried about is the rest of the claims, the ones that have already raised red flags."

Vlad grinds his teeth. "Shit happens."

"I hate mistakes—especially if I deem them avoidable. You have been sloppy. As a result, you have drawn too much attention to our business."

His face is turning beet red.

"And one more thing," she adds, as cool as can be. "The business is facing an increased risk of being exposed as a fraud. Therefore, this was not the right time to get rid of that woman, Linda—despite all her faults."

Vlad makes a show of flicking some dust off his shoulder. "What's done is done."

"Well." She huffs. "Now what do I do?"

He points at me. "I brought you this one in her place."

In nearly every way, I'm a stand-in for Linda. Everything I wear—the black sweater, the skirt with silver buttons down the front, even the footwear—all belong to the deceased. Her smoky smell, infused in every fiber of her clothing, wraps over me. I can't shake it off, nor can I escape a sudden sense of loss. When Linda was alive, I never felt for her—but now I find myself reflecting on her suffering. Her pain was so palpable as she drew her last breath.

Vlad nudges me. "Hey, I have just introduced you. Why are you so silent?"

Turning to his accomplice, I try for a confident, cheery tone, in stark contrast to what's in my heart. "Hello there!"

Mrs. Komarov looks me up and down, as if I were a piece of merchandise. "Well, can she read? Is she smart enough to analyze data? And most importantly, can she lie with a straight face?"

Vlad curls his lips just short of a smirk. "I bet she can, especially when her life depends on it. Why not give her a try?"

"I will." The old woman shakes her head in dismay. "But it goes against my better judgment."

"It does? Why?"

"I just happened to overhear your little chitchat, Vlad."

"And?"

"I do not trust her. She makes you talk too much."

"Fine! From now on, she is in your hands."

"As she should be." The old woman presses a cold finger under my chin, lifts it, studies my face under the electric light.

Vlad lets out a sigh. "Well?"

"Well." She lets go of me and takes a step back. "I do not like what I see in her eyes."

"Oh, that's silly. What is it you see?"

"Fire."

"What?" He waves a hand in dismissal. "Not sure I understand you."

She spits. "Not sure you want to understand."

"Mamushka darling, here is what I do get," he says, with disdain. "You hate this one as much as you hated Linda—or, for that matter, any other woman that happened to cross paths with me."

"Granted, this one is a pretty little thing. Perhaps," says the old woman, with a ring of disgust, "you have a soft spot in your heart for her?"

"No," says Vlad, much too quickly. "Everyone knows I am as hard as I ever was."

He thrusts his chest forward and pounds a fist against it, which does nothing to impress her. Mrs. Komarov sets her hands on her hips and pleats her brow, straining to read him. "In that case," she says acidly, "it must be just plain lust."

Vlad seems determined to stand up to her scrutiny. His expression remains unchanged.

She pulls a bit of warmth into her voice and, at the same time, clutches his arm tightly with her bony fingers. "Remember our old place, back in London? Remember the apple tree that stood in our front garden?"

He squirms out of her grip. "Vaguely."

Mrs. Komarov clicks her tongue. "Nah, how could you forget that tree? The day you left for Moscow, it burned to the ground—"

"You don't say. What about it?"

"Planning a fraud is much like that tree—"

"Oh, stop right there! *Please* spare me this so-called wisdom of yours! I have no patience for comparing my business to some god-forsaken tree."

In a snap, her voice goes back to cold. "You must tend to it. You must sustain a steady growth. You must exterminate its parasites. You must monitor the root system so it can have a firm grip on the dirt and, in time, shoot out some limbs. And after all that time, all that investment—just when it starts yielding its best fruit—that's when someone like her comes along, strikes a match, and with a little flickering flame, turns the whole thing to ashes."

Chapter 21

Plodding past Vlad and his men—all of whom have turned somewhat stiff in her presence—Mrs. Komarov takes my arm with a firm hand. Boy, is she irresistible—and not in a good way! She pushes me into the back room. It has a narrow exit door, barred by a heavy-duty, all-steel door lock, and no windows. As the pale fluorescent light reveals, it is in some disarray.

A man's jacket is flung in a heap, along with a frayed scarf, on the ripped vinyl seat of a metal chair. Another chair—balancing on its two front legs with its hind ones up in the air—leans forward against a large desk laden with stacks and stacks of disheveled papers. Some notes carry smudges that look and smell like cigarette ash. One of them has slipped to the linoleum floor. It has come to a rest, crumpled, bearing the dull mark of a shoe.

"Sit," the old woman tells me. "I hope my son didn't tell you anything about me?"

"Only good things," I say.

Her face registers an odd mixture of relief and disappointment. Mrs. Komarov mutters to herself that Vlad should know better than to engage in useless chitchat. Friends should be chosen with as much mindfulness as enemies. He should keep his mouth shut about his family in general and his darling Mamushka in particular.

From there, she pivots into a long and convoluted explanation, which I can barely follow, and for a good reason. When overtaken by anger, she starts rambling. At this point, English words fail her, and she resorts to Russian.

At any rate, the old woman goes on and on about the work I must do: sort out some medical codes and figure a way to correct the stupid billing mistakes made by whomever they employed before me. Of course, *employed* is used quite loosely here. I suspect *coerced* is more to the point. Or even *forced*.

I nod. "Sure, Mrs. Komarov, I can do all that—but first, I need to go to the bathroom. Badly."

With a little frown, she points a knuckled finger at the corner of the room, where a narrow door stands slightly ajar.

I get in and close the door. Just as expected, it can't be locked from the inside. A wastebasket, overflowing with dirty tissues, peeks out from the corner. Above the yellow-ringed toilet there is a small window, its casement thrown open to let out the stink. To my disappointment, escaping is out of the question. It is barred.

I hear her footfalls pacing to and fro on the other side of the door, and her voice, somewhat muffled, calling out, "Whatever you do, just be quick! Do not make me wait."

Confused and dejected, I desperately need some private time. I have to collect my wits. How can I distract her so she lets me be—if only for a few moments?

I produce some noise by flushing the toilet a couple of times, then running the faucet for a bit. Meanwhile, I take Michael's cellphone out of its hiding place—inside the double-knot between the sleeves of the sweater—and, hoping to contact him as well as the police, I switch it on.

A text flashes for a split second—*Don't worry, sweetheart. I know where they're taking you*—before the screen goes black.

Oh no! I wish I had the charger with me.

Now what?

Dumbfounded, I stare at the cellphone, breathing *Don't worry, sweetheart* over and again. I taste these words, roll them on my tongue this way and that, each one separately and all of them together. And I wonder: at what point during my ordeal did Michael text them to me? The answer is crucial. It may offer a glimmer of hope—or let me lose it altogether.

I know where they're taking you.

Did he write that when I was flown aboard the helicopter to UCLA Medical Center, where Linda's body was deposited along with my ID cards? Her death was reported as mine, so at that point, Michael might have turned around. Stricken with grief, he might have headed back home to break the sad news to my parents. At my moment of need, are they wasting time, mourning my untimely demise?

I know where they're taking you.

Did Michael write it later, when I was driven in Vlad's van to this very place? If so, there is a chance that my rescue effort has not been aborted. He may still be on his way. Is he standing outside the entrance door, about to break in and save me?

I tie the sleeves into a double knot, securing the cellphone in it. Having draped the sweater casually around my shoulders, I open the narrow door. Mrs. Komarov stands there, hands on her hips, looking me squarely in the eye. She taps her foot impatiently and in no uncertain terms, demands, "Give me that thing, right now!"

"Thing?" My tone sounds as innocent as can be. I add a note of hurt, just for good measure. "What thing?"

Despite my calm appearance, fear gnaws at me. Has the old woman guessed, somehow, that I'm concealing a cellphone? If so, I'll have to point out that it is a useless thing, nothing more than a piece of plastic, its charge depleted.

I adjust the black sweater over my shoulders and flash a tearful smile at her.

To my surprise, Mrs. Komarov reaches below my chest and then lower still, all the way down the side of my skirt—well, Linda's skirt, actually. The dearly departed won't need it ever again. In a snap, the old woman rips a slightly crumpled cigarette box out of my pocket.

"No smoking in here," she grumbles.

Which makes me wonder what else may be tucked in that pocket, courtesy of the deceased. A matchbox? A lighter?

My pulse begins pounding. Hard.

Can the old woman hear the drumbeat of my heart? A sudden battle cry roars in my head, shaking my whole being. Can she discern it? As I'm under her watchful eye, I can't act on it. I can't reach into that pocket and search for something that—in a pinch—may serve as a weapon.

Mrs. Komarov opens the cigarette box, fishes out the lone Camel, and sticks it between her lips. Then, she thrusts out her hand and demands, "Out, out with the rest of it! Don't make me search you."

I stuff my fingers in the pocket and feel a cold, metallic thing. A lighter. What choice do I have but to place it on her palm?

Meanwhile, lining the very bottom of that pocket is another object, probably a matchbook. It is thin enough to be ignored, which of course I do. For now.

Mrs. Komarov presses her thumb on the spark-wheel and lights the Camel. Inhaling deeply, she takes a step back. "I told that *mudak*—I mean, that asshole, Linda—a thousand times. No Smoking."

"I had no idea—"

"*Ti Durak!*" She spits. "You are a moron."

"Sorry."

"An empty head is not what I need!"

Despite the insults, I bend over backwards to sound agreeable. "What is it you need, Mrs. Komarov?"

The old woman grabs me by the ear and forces me to the chair. "Sit. Go over the paperwork. Figure out what the hell is wrong. Why are these insurance companies on my back? How do I shake them off?"

The desk is littered with paper. Given this clutter, the work asked of me seems doomed to failure. Some of the letters have yellowed already. Some have somewhat ragged edges and carry an accidental cigarette hole, burnt all the way through. And on others, the ink is smudged.

I sort the documents into two piles. In one, complaints from beneficiaries. In the other, inquiries initiated by this or that insurance company: Health Net, United Healthcare, Humana, MedNet, and others. The complaints and inquiries have one thing in common: they all question the referenced billing charges. The clinics that issued these charges are fake, I suspect. And the professionals employed by them must all be make-believe persons, constructed out of stolen identities.

What catches my attention is the mismatch between the stated medical specialty of these so-called professionals and the codes used to bill patients for their services. It's almost comical: eye doctors billed for bladder tests, ear, nose and throat specialists billed for pregnancy ultrasounds, obstetricians for skin allergies, and dermatologists for heart exams.

This is so similar to the news story I discussed with Pa recently. Ten years ago, a ring of criminals called the Armenian Power set up a similar scheme. They used fake clinics and identity theft to file fraudulent claims, bilking Medicare out of over a hundred million dollars. Eventually, the FBI caught them, simply because of a clerical mismatch—much like what's here—between medical specialties and billing codes.

"Mrs. Komarov," I say, raising my eyes to her. "The devil is in the details."

"Huh? What does that mean?"

"It means, someone in your organization came up with questionable methods of pulling off this fraud, which he must have learned, one way or another, from his involvement in the Armenian Power."

The old woman doesn't even ask what the *Armenian Power* might be. She knows. Pursing her cracked lips, she says nothing for a long while. At last, she throws the cigarette butt to the floor and mashes it to ashes with her shoe.

"You're right," she mutters. "I see I will have to be completely frank with you."

"Please do."

"The man you're talking about is Oleg's brother. He joined us as soon as he got out of prison—"

"Oh? And I thought every member of that gang is still behind bars."

"No," she corrects me. "Not anymore. Because of the coronavirus, some inmates such as that guy have become eligible for early release."

So I've heard. Lately, early release has been a controversial topic. Some in the public see it as the humanitarian thing to do during these troubled times. Others deem it downright dangerous.

Of course, there are certain criteria for early release, set by the Corrections Department. For example, the inmates must be presently incarcerated at institutions that house large populations of high-risk patients. Also, they must not be incarcerated for domestic violence or other violent crime.

"So," I say, "when Oleg's brother was let loose, he joined your organization?"

"Exactly," she says. "He brought with him the expertise we needed."

"Can I talk to him?"

"No. He died."

"Oh?"

"For him, freedom came too late," says Mrs. Komarov. "The virus killed him a couple of weeks after his release, which gave us little time to extract the idea for his fraud scheme out of him."

"Too bad."

Over the rim of her glasses, the old woman hangs her eyes on me, this time with newfound appreciation. "Obviously, the idea was clever, but the execution—sloppy, which we didn't immediately catch."

"That," I daresay, "was your mistake."

The old woman spits. "Indeed. I realize it now."

"It's going to take you down—"

"Unless," she cuts in, "you can tell me what needs to be fixed."

Just then, a sudden commotion. Some shouts erupt in the main space of the so-called clinic, along with a sound of clapping.

Vlad's head pops in. "See?" he cries, shaking an envelope in his fist. "The mailman just delivered a check, the first check from one of the insurance companies!"

"Really?"

"Really! Didn't I tell you there's nothing to worry about?"

The old woman shakes her head. "About that, son, you're wrong."

His icy-blue eyes shine brightly, glazing the emptiness within. "Soon, more checks will come pouring in. You will see!"

"How much is the check for?"

"Forty thousand dollars."

"Well," says Mrs. Komarov. "That is what I call *a good beginning!*"

"Just so, Mamushka!"

Swept by his excitement, Mrs. Komarov gets to her feet and hurries out the door to join the others, leaving me behind. On her way out she says, over her shoulder, "You, stay put. I need you to come up with a solution. Work on it like your life depends on it."

I do. First—as soon as she turns her back to me—a quick change of clothes. I take off Linda's shoes because by now my feet are killing me and remove the black skirt because it's a bit tight. I look good in my spandex leggings, if I say so myself.

Then I smooth down the side of the skirt, sliding my hand into the pocket and grabbing the matchbook. Nearly all of its matches are gone. Only a single one is left. I'll have to make it count.

With trembling fingers, I tear it out of the matchbook and strike it against the rough narrow strip. It doesn't ignite. I strike again, approach the wastebasket, which is set in the corner behind the toilet, and throw it there, burning.

The flame is flimsy, at first.

For a while, I believe it has been extinguished. The match has sunk out of sight and disappeared under the dirty tissues. Then, a subtle glow appears. A little tongue of fire starts licking, touching a corner of a tissue here, an edge there, slithering across the mess, consuming it hungrily.

Once the fire starts blazing through the wastebasket itself, I carry the flaming thing, set it under the desk, heap in handfuls of the oldest billing complaints, and hurry out the door. I close it shut behind me and, with a little cheer, join the others in their impromptu celebration.

Soon, all of us will feel the heat.

Chapter 22

If anyone would ask me later why I threw a match into a wastebasket full of tissues, added a pile of the papers I was supposed to be organizing, and left it behind a closed door, burning, I would be hard pressed to explain my plan. Why? Because I have none. Impulse is what drives me. The events of the last couple of days have forced my hand. I can no longer remain inactive.

By instinct, I grasp that something drastic needs to happen—for better or worse—to change my situation. Fire will do. Things staying as they are will only prolong my misery.

The celebration has just gotten underway in the main space. Hearing the hoots and the chest beating, I sneak out of the back room to watch the gang up-close.

Colorful confetti—leftover from the out-of-business party store that used to rent this space—is being tossed all around. Vlad himself is blasting out one party popper after another with unbridled delight.

His men, too, are in a festive mood. A bit tipsy already, they crowd around the long table, now covered by a paper tablecloth. Mrs. Komarov stands at the head of the table, ladling cold Russian soup from a large plastic container into plastic bowls for all of them. From here, it smells a bit like sour milk.

"Thank you, thank you!" says the first in line, having gulped it down hungrily. "What a delicious Okroshka, with boiled potatoes and raw radishes and cucumbers. Just like my mother used to make."

She gloats over the compliment. "More food yet to come," she says, with a matronly smile.

Some of the men set crates of beer at Vlad's feet, others—pour drinks over his head. The anointment is rowdy, but Vlad seems to bask in it.

I notice that the main door has been unlatched, perhaps to bring in the food. This is my chance to flee—if not for Mrs. Komarov. She is the first to notice that I've slipped out of the back room.

"Why are you here?" she demands, gruffly. "Did I not tell you to stay put? Your job is to figure out how I can shake the damn insurance companies off my back—"

"Ah, stop it, Mamushka," says Vlad. His British accent makes that single Russian word sound out of place.

"No," she counters, shaking the ladle in his face. "You stop!"

He claps a hand around my waist and pulls me to his chest. His mouth reeks of cheap beer. "Let her join us! What's a party without a beautiful woman?"

Her face reddens. She grabs my arm angrily and wrenches me from his hold.

Her eyes blazing, she tells him, "*Zacroy rot!*"

"Shut up? Me?" Vlad gnashes his teeth. "How can you even say that especially now, when everyone here celebrates my success? Don't you see, I am on top of the world?"

Mrs. Komarov gnashes her teeth, way louder than he did. If this were a competition, she would get the gold. "Without me, you will hit rock bottom before you know it. So, pay respect. Do not dare cut in when I am talking. And I mean, ever!"

He wipes off beads of sweat from his brow. "Forgive me, Mamushka."

At this point, the old woman does something I haven't expected of her. Shooting a victorious glare at him, she sets away the ladle and opens her arms. He submits to her hug.

Then she turns to me. "And you—do I have to repeat myself? Why did you not stay put, like I told you?"

"Mrs. Komarov," I say, struggling to come up with some excuse. "I think I know how to correct those clerical mistakes."

She spits. "You do, do you?"

"Yes," I lie. "And if I'm right, you can resubmit the corrected billing to the insurance companies. You can explain you got things wrong in the first try."

She scratches her head. "Like we say in Russian, '*The first pancake is always lumpy.*'"

"Exactly. Go for the second try. The insurance companies will approve the changes and stop bothering you. But first, I need to learn a few details from you—which is why I've come in to look for you."

"A few details? Such as what?"

"Such as, which insurance company sent you this check for forty thousand dollars?"

"MedNet."

I ask, "Can I see their letter? It would help to learn what was done right in this particular case, as opposed to the other ones."

Vlad checks his breast pocket, fetches the letter, hands it to me.

I raise it to my eyes, barely able to focus, unsure where to go next. So, I drag out the words, "Ah-huh! Just as I thought—"

The old woman asks, "What?"

And Vlad echoes, "What?"

And just as I open my mouth to say, "Well, you see," the main door opens and Oleg steps in. He has been standing guard outside all this time. "Vy is it so hot in here?"

Mrs. Komarov claps her hands. "All because of Vlad! He is such a hotshot!"

"Yes," says Oleg, with a wink. "But vee all know who is boss!"

Vlad frowns. "Get out, get out right now, Oleg! You should stay on the lookout—"

"And miss party? No vay!"

Meanwhile behind him, someone else pops in. He wears a mask over his mouth and nose and a blue visor cap with a Dominoes Pizza logo on his head, so I don't immediately recognize him, and neither does anyone else. In his hand is an insulated pizza delivery bag.

"Who ordered pizza?" asks Vlad.

And Oleg says, "Who cares? Food! Let's eat—"

"No!" Vlad raises his hand, and everyone stops cheering. "I mean, really. Who ordered the damn thing?"

"Hey," says the delivery boy, holding out his hand. "All I want is my tip, is all."

Out of the blue, Mrs. Komarov starts shrieking. The need to hear me explain about medical codes, mismanaged charges, and billing procedures seems to have flown right out of her head, for which I'm thankful.

"Oh no!" she cries. "No, no, no!"

The delivery boy shrugs. "What, no tip?"

"Look!" The flesh jiggles under her arm as she points a knuckled finger at the window. "Cops!"

Indeed, three police cars have just come to a grinding halt at the opposite side of the street. For now, no one has filed out of them, or so it seems.

As quickly as her feet would allow her, the old woman backs away. Tying a babushka over her head, she trudges towards the inner door, the one leading to the back room and to its barred exit door. She is followed by most of the gang—except for two.

Besieged by the empty crates at his feet, his head glistening with rivulets of sticky beer, and his shoulders sprinkled with shiny confetti, Vlad remains stuck in place. He pleats his forehead, as if asking himself what the hell has just happened. Then, perhaps in search for the culprit, he raises his eyes and looks me in the eye.

"My darling Mamushka is right," he says, darkly. "She always is."

Meanwhile, Oleg seems to be in no hurry to either hide or escape. He snatches the pizza bag from the delivery boy and unzips it. A puff of steam rises out of it, but the cheesy aroma is tinged with another smell. It is subtle, but to me—unmistakable.

Smoke.

It seeps out slowly, steadily at the far end of the space, under the inner door. Am I the only one to detect it?

Mrs. Komarov stops midway to the back room and casts a look through the window at the police, filing out of their vehicles. Clearly, she is focused on them and not on any other danger. She calls her son to come over, to hide with her from the cops. Some of the gangsters parrot her calls, but Vlad waves them all away.

Facing me, Oleg stuffs a huge slice of pizza in his mouth. Chewing and chomping greedily, he staggers out the door. His shadowy figure is still visible through the window—until he disappears behind one of the cars, somewhere around the street corner.

"Hey, where's everybody going?" asks the delivery boy. "And who's going to pay me?"

"Here is what's coming to you," says Vlad. He clenches his fist and without further ado, knocks him off his feet. The blue visor cap with the Dominoes Pizza logo rolls onto the floor.

Oh my, it's Michael!

While he rolls to his knees, Vlad steps on his hand.

Michael yells—I cringe, feeling his pain—grabs Vlad's ankle with his free hand and pulls him down, hard.

Rolling on the dusty floor, Vlad kicks him in the ribs. Michael folds in agony. I throw myself at Vlad, scratch his shoulder all the way down to his elbow till it bleeds.

Vlad clutches my wrist, forces me into the corner, and hisses in my ear, "Ashley Winters, did you call the cops on me?"

"No—"

"Oh, why do I even bother?" Vlad slaps my face so hard that it makes my skin burn. "I always knew you can lie with a straight face. Especially when your life depends on it."

I try to wriggle away from him, but slip over the confetti strewn around. Vlad kneels by my side, puts his knee between my legs, and leans closer, his hand clamping my throat. And while my windpipe is pressed—while I'm fighting for air—he mutters, between clenched teeth, "Mamushka knows best."

The last thing I see before my lights go out is Michael, punching him in the face.

*

The first thing I hear when I regain consciousness is his voice. "Oh please, sweetheart," Michael murmurs. "Please, wake up."

I find myself in his arms. His touch feels so good. I'm so happy he's here. At last, I'm not alone. But other than his face, I barely recognize anything else around us. Vlad is nowhere to be seen and, in the span of a few seconds, the entire space has fallen into chaos.

I've thought that *all hell breaks loose* is an exaggerated figure of speech—until this moment. I see the old woman reaching to grab the handle, which must be scorchingly hot to the touch. With a sudden grunt, she tears open the inner door, then shakes her hand, shakes it fervently. It must hurt like hell.

A roaring fire blows in her face. It seems almost human, the way it bends over as if to smell her hair, taste the sleeves of her dress, the hem.

In utter shock, Mrs. Komarov stumbles backward, one step, two. Falling to the ground, she screams in terror, and the flames recoil for a second before bursting out at her even brighter than before.

Meanwhile, the first cop comes in. Others follow, weapons drawn. The gangsters step over Mrs. Komarov and over each other in a mad rush to flee. Confusion sets in as they scatter every which way, unclear where to go: away from the blaze—or away from the police?

Michael and I make our way through hissing smoke to save the old woman. We peer at the scene between one tongue of fire and another. A hairy leg is spotted here, an arm there, and on occasion—*Voola*—a snake, tattooed around an elbow.

I suck in a deep breath and duck through the flame in search of Mrs. Komarov. I'm guided by her frantic shrieks as a burning beam has collapsed next to her. Her babushka, now removed from her head, is now held with her quivering fingers, covering her mouth and nose from the smoke. We grab her arms and drag her together step by step around the overturned table, across a puddle of spilled Okroshka soup, and out to the street, where an ambulance has just arrived.

We carry her past the cops who surround the place and past the firefighters who are setting up their equipment. The old woman complains, her voice scratchy from smoke inhalation, about the stinging in her eyes.

Medics arrive. They apply medication over the burn on her right side to relieve the pain. They also suggest we get tested for COVID-19.

"Oh no," says Mrs. Komarov. "I heard all about the nasal swab test."

One of the medics explains, "It captures a lot of viral material concentrated in the back of the nose—"

"It is notoriously unpleasant." She coughs. "You are not going to stick that thing up my nose!"

"No worries. We offer also a saliva test. It's easy. All you have to do is spit into a sterilized container, which is then sent to the lab for processing. The results will be available in a few hours."

"Fine. Spitting I like."

Strangely, the one person missing through all of this is her son. For a second, I think I see him across the street, watching us. A sudden rush of adrenaline sends me dashing over there, ready to point him out for the cops—only to realize there's no one there. What I saw must have been a phantom of imagination, a dance of flames.

My tie-dyed undershirt is drenched with sweat. Even so, I fall into Michael's hug. His face is covered with smoky soot, and so is mine—but no matter. We cling together for dear life.

The medic turns his attention to us. While being treated for our injuries, we exchange a glance. Even without words, I know what Michael is asking me.

Has Vlad perished in the fire?

Chapter 23

I would later learn that some of the gangsters fled—with police in hot pursuit—as far as the outskirts of the city. Local residents, who had been alerted, nabbed a few of them, including Oleg.

In my deposition, I state that he is the one who raped me, all these months ago. I feel relieved, at long last, that he is going to rot in jail for that and for his other crimes. But the leader of the pack, Vlad, is still at large.

Not far from the so-called dermatology clinic, which is now fully engulfed in flames, my Escape has been collecting dust since last night. It looks funny, leaning heavily over its front rims, its tires slashed. Normally, I'd let Michael replace it, but once he positions the jack beneath the frame of the vehicle, I catch him wincing in pain. So I ask him to step aside. And while he's complaining that I'm making him feel useless, and it isn't fair, and so on, I do the rest myself.

"Take it easy, love. You've done enough for one day," I say. "If not for you, I'd end up being Vlad's slave for life."

I rejoice in my newfound freedom. And in spite of my own injuries, doing physical work makes me feel—oh, I don't know—elated? Invincible? I loosen the lug nuts a bit, then crank the jack, lifting the vehicle until the slashed tire is six inches above ground.

Michael gives me a sidelong glance. "Nice leggings."

"I prefer jeans, but had to give them up." I unscrew the lug nuts. "Don't even ask. Long story."

He keeps looking while I remove the tire, mount the spare on the lug bolts, tighten the nuts and finally, lower the Escape.

From time to time, a shadow stirs across the street. Maybe it's just Michael's reflection in the opposite store window, or mine. A spark strays away from the spectacular shower of cinders raining down a short distance away. It flies, flipping in the air over the flaming storefronts.

We're ready, oh so ready to go. If Vlad is anywhere near, we need to avoid him like the plague.

We head to Laguna Beach, stopping only once in a Shell gas station. While Michael fills the gas tank, I go to the bathroom and scrub my hands and face vigorously, like I'm preparing to perform some surgery. The soapy water spins into the sink drain. With a little slurp, nothing is left but a trace of foam. Sadness wells in my chest. I want to wash it away, scour the memory of my ordeal. I want to have a good cry and move on. But I can't.

It doesn't feel like it's over.

I go back to the car, lower the windows to let out the smell of smoke, emanating from our clothing and hair. Then I start the engine. It sputters on occasion, but no matter. On the way, Michael fills me in on the essential details of what happened at his end, starting at the point of his return home from the hospital.

The Nixle alert notified him that Los Angeles County Sheriff's Helicopter was on its way to Pirates' Cove, but the idea that it was dispatched for my sake did not occur to him. Only when Rita's email reached him did Michael put two and two together. She told him to get in touch with me by calling his own own cellphone number. He promised to come to my help, one way or another.

For Michael, driving a car was out of the question, not only because his Tesla had been burnt by the gang but because he was on pain killers, as his shoulder was still hurting around the site of the removed bullet. Ignoring doctors' orders to take things easy, he called an Uber cab and set out to Los Angeles to save me.

His directions were based on tracking the GPS readout of his own cellphone, which I carried on me at all times, knowing it was my connection to him, my lifeline.

Of course, he considered the chance that the cellphone was taken from me and attached to someone else, a decoy. Accepting that possibility would have left him clueless, so Michael decided to disregard it. He monitored the readout doggedly, praying that in the end, it would lead him to where I was.

Then came an announcement on the car radio. It said that in the aftermath of the helicopter rescue operation, a young woman was delivered to UCLA Medical Center. She was pronounced dead. Her identity was not disclosed, but the circumstances suggested it was me.

"I was afraid of that," I say. "Afraid you'd give up on me, as soon as you heard that news."

And Michael admits, "I almost did."

I can't help but ask, "What stopped you, then?"

"A good cry."

"A good cry?" I envy him for that, for the ease he has with his feelings. "That never worked for me, never did anything except leave me emotionally wrung out."

"Just the words I was looking for. Wrung out. Stricken by the most daunting sense of loss. I struggled to think straight, wiped my eyes over and again, but tears…" His voice falters. "Tears kept coming. Everything around me looked blurry—except for one thing: the GPS readout. To my amazement, the cellphone was still on the move, still changing position!"

Michael lets out a smile, then turns serious again. "So, I weighed the odds. Would a killer take his victim's cellphone, at the risk of being tracked? That made little sense to me. What seemed more reasonable was the idea that you survived, that someone else had been delivered to UCLA Medical Center in your place."

Michael turns silent for a while. The medics that cleaned his face must have missed a spot: the side of his nose is still smeared with ash. And his shoulder must be in pain again, as he presses a hand around it.

I'm tempted to get off the road and find us a place where we can snuggle, where I can kiss away his hurt and be kissed back in return. Instead, I grit my teeth. I must drive on, must go see my parents, because only then will they trust I'm out of trouble. It is this urgency—as well as longing for my dog, Browny—that keeps my hands on the steering wheel.

"The idea that you're still alive persisted in my head," Michael says. "With all my heart, I hoped it was more than merely wishful thinking. I hoped it was the truth."

"How did you figure out where they were taking me?"

"Oh, that was a calculated guess," he says. "Your friend, Rita, told me about the fake clinic, about your visit there last night and what you found. So, when the GPS readout showed you getting closer and closer to that address, I made a run for it."

"Thank God for intuition!"

"Thank God for persistence, too! I alerted the Los Angeles County Sheriff's office. At first, they wouldn't believe me. To them, the story seemed far-fetched."

"No wonder," I mutter. "They know you as a software hacker, often working around the edges of what is considered lawful."

His eyes shine. He accepts what I've said as if it were a badge of honor. "To them, I'm a rebel."

"So, why would they trust anything you have to tell them?"

"They didn't. But then—once they checked with UCLA Medical Center, and the identity of the dead woman was called into question—they started to pay attention."

*

Having arrived at Laguna Beach, I park the Escape and hop out. Barely able to curb my excitement, I climb the uneven stone walkway leading up to Pa's front deck. Meanwhile, Michael waits behind for me.

I remind myself to keep a distance from my father when we meet—even more than the officially recommended six feet away. I must avoid contact with him, because of having spent time in a confined space with the gangsters, including Linda, who was coughing, and Oleg, whose brother was released from prison only to succumb to the virus.

Contagion is the last thing we need. All I want is to set eyes on Pa from afar and let him see that I'm all right. After that, I plan to send him an air-kiss, wave goodnight, and take Browny with me.

Clinging to the hill, Pa's one-bedroom rental seems more tilted in silhouette, more dilapidated. There is no light in the window, even though I've left a message on his phone to let him know I'm coming. My heart skips a beat. Something is wrong.

"Hello! Pa?" I cry, wiping my feet on the welcome mat, then taking a few steps back, out of an abundance of caution.

No one answers.

Why isn't Browny barking? I've been missing him so much and expected him to leap over me and lick my face all over. Why isn't Pa answering the doorbell? I've prepared myself to stop him from coming out to greet me, arms wide open.

Maybe he's out walking the dog. Should I wait for his return?

I shout, "Anybody home?"

Again, nothing.

No sound is heard, other than the slight rustle of shrubs at the edge of the deck. Their branches frame a night view of the Pacific Ocean, glinting out there, shimmering in the moonlight.

A shadow rises from the bench, and now I see a man's outline. At first I think it's my father, but then realize my mistake. It's Vlad.

My throat tightens. My vocal cords fail me. For the life of me, I can't produce a single sound.

He takes a step closer, clapping a hand over my mouth to prevent me from crying out, which I can't do anyway. But I struggle. I try in vain to hit him in the groin before he subdues me.

"Oh, what fun." Vlad takes a deep breath, then kicks in the door, which shows me how brazen he is. He throws me inside. "This visit won't take long, I promise."

I detect a note of something in that voice, but can't quite place it. Vengeance?

The hair rises on my goosebumps. I shiver. For a split second, I spot a metallic flash. His knife.

In the dark interior, I scramble to my feet. I tumble over to the kitchenette, drag my hands frantically across the counter. It is dotted by some objects. My touch gives me only a vague idea of what they are. I perk my ears, hoping to hear the clink of cutlery. But no, just some dull noise of plastic utensils and the swish of paper plates. Nothing I can use against him.

He rolls the words in that British accent of his, which is so familiar, and yet so terribly startling.

"My dear," says Vlad. "This is the last time I wait for you."

Chapter 24

"So, are you ready to spend your last moments with me? I promise not to disappoint." Vlad leans over me from behind, his left arm tightening around my waist, his right elbow resting over the tip of my shoulder so as to steady his wrist, his control of the knife.

I try to swing my arm back and hit him, which only serves to make his grip more painful.

"What is the point of resisting me? Give it up, will you? I'm going to tell you a little story." Vlad gives me one rough shake after another, which brings me to the verge of fainting.

When I come to, he presses on. "Long ago, when I was a child, my mother used to be a seamstress. I would watch her pluck pins out of the pincushion and mark the design on the fabric."

His story sounds nostalgic, at first—but I know it is a prelude for a kill.

Next to my ear, he's grinding his teeth. "Oh, how I hated her customers for nudging her to hurry! How I hated her for bowing down before them like a common servant! All for a few meager rubles. I was embarrassed by it. Infuriated."

I say not a word, as I recall him sharing a childhood memory with Linda before slitting her throat.

"By the way my darling Mamushka averted her eyes from me, she probably knew how I felt," he says, his voice cracking. "But she never acknowledged my hurt; never shared her own. Instead, she focused only on the stitch, on executing it with absolute precision. In a barely audible hiss, she would quote this Russian proverb, which has guided my hand ever since. *'Measure seven times, cut once.'*"

I can't see his smile—but feel it, somehow, at my back, leaching into my flesh, sinking into my bones. He lets the blade hover over the base of my neck, barely coming into contact, barely imparting its cold touch.

"For you," says Vlad, "I am willing to take things real slow, real gentle—not like I did with Linda."

With effort, I find my voice. "Let me go."

"Later." He scores my skin, ever so lightly. "This is going to be real easy. Like slicing through butter."

Hoping someone out there would hear me, I scream at the top of my lungs.

Vlad draws in a deep breath, which tells me how aroused he is, preparing for the slash. Just then, a sudden noise outside catches our attention. My body trembles; his shakes.

"What the hell was that?" he asks.

And now, here is that sound again, only louder. A second rock hits the window, this one busting it wide open, shards of glass sent spinning across the floor, one of them catching a dim ray of light.

Caught by surprise, Vlad inadvertently loosens his hold on me for a second, which is time enough for me to slip out of it, fall to my knees, and grasp the sharp fragment from the floor—at long last, a weapon!—which I slam, with all the power I can muster, right into his foot.

Yowling, he folds over. He tries to take a step, but the shard pins him in place. Tearing his foot away would free him—at the cost of cutting open the wound and causing even more damage. In torment, Vlad seems to have no courage for that.

Just in case he manages to muster it, I crawl away as fast as I can. Hands bleeding, I gather more glass splinters from the floor so if he comes after me, I can use them to fight him off.

Meanwhile, a sharp clinking sound bursts out, which is music to my ears. One figure—Pa—clears the jugged edges from the moonlit windowsill, and another—Michael—hops in.

Stuck in place, Vlad growls. "Damnit! Not you again—"

"My thoughts exactly," says Pa.

They know each other from years ago, when Vlad took over my father's job at Southern California Edison. For the sake of a smooth transition, the company made Pa train his successor before laying him off. So, no love lost there.

Vlad twists his body away from Pa and throws his knife at Michael—only to miss him.

"Easy now," says Michael. He picks the knife from the floor and casts it to the far corner, clear out of Vlad's reach.

Vlad doesn't remain empty-handed. His weapon of choice is gone, but his fingers are already fluttering over his handgun holster, just short of grabbing his Russian M1895 Nagant revolver.

I regret not paying attention to it earlier. I should have reached for the weapon when I had the chance.

"I wouldn't use that if I were you," says Michael. "This place is completely surrounded by police."

Vlad cries, "Liar!"

"Maybe I am and maybe I'm not. Want to bet?"

Vlad hesitates—but Michael doesn't. He pushes the Russian to the floor and throw himself on top of him. Glass cracks under them as they exchange blows, and—*boom!*—a shot rattles the air.

Some powder starts falling from the ceiling, where a bullet has nicked the paint. It takes me a minute to realize that Michael is alive, that he is the victor, having wrenched the revolver from his opponent's hand.

Michael picks himself up and dusts off his knees while Vlad remains spread eagle on the floor, his foot bleeding profusely.

Will he ask forgiveness for his attempt on my life or at least say something eloquent to explain it? Well, not exactly. He props himself up on his elbows, then catches his breath long enough to grumble. "Oh fuck."

Pa says, "Whoa. That's a nasty wound."

"Courtesy of your darling daughter," says Vlad, his tone acid.

Pa brings a bandage from his medicine cabinet. "Try to lie still. The medics are on their way."

"The hell with them. The hell with you, too."

Between one pained breath and another, Vlad fixes his eyes on me. I expect to see the usual emptiness. Instead, I find hate.

"I made the mistake to bring that bitch into my organization, even though Mamushka told me not to, and see where it got me," he says, with such disdain in his voice that I shudder. "She burned down my business. She took me down for all I'm worth."

Pa shrugs. "Can't say I'm sorry to hear it."

Michael unloads the revolver, gives me a smile. "Neither can I."

Despite feeling shaky, I rise to my feet even before he offers me his hand.

Two cops burst through the door, followed by paramedics.

"That's it," Vlad says, his voice whiny. "My life is over."

And I say, "Better yours than mine."

Michael hands me the cellphone, fully charged now, and I call Ma to tell her not to worry, I'm fine, just a bit tired, nothing serious, really, let's talk later, when I've had a chance to rest.

During the drive to Michael's place—after Vlad was placed in handcuffs and led away to the police car—I get the results of our COVID-19 saliva tests. I've been worried about my health and the health of those close to me ever since I spent time with Linda, who kept coughing in my face, and with Oleg, whose brother succumbed to the virus shortly after his release from prison.

But as it turns out, my fears have been unfounded. The test results are negative. I'm not infectious, and neither is Michael. I listen to the rush of air from my lungs as I let out a sigh of relief.

Still, my muscles feel tense. I tell myself that my ordeal is over, but find myself unable to fully comprehend it.

Once in Michael's home, I collapse into his leather armchair and rest my feet on the footstool. It's nearly midnight. Instead of turning on the light, Michael sets a couple of thick candles on the mantle. Eyes half open, I try to relax by their soft glow.

Browny is lying at my feet, panting. From time to time he gives a little whine. Perhaps he's disappointed for being left out of all the fun. Michael has already told me how he spotted my father walking the dog just past the Escape; how both of them saw a figure rising from the bench on the front porch; how they realized it must have been Vlad; how they concluded he was about to kill me; how they called 911; and how they left Browny behind, in the vehicle, so his barks wouldn't spoil the element of surprise when both of them barged in through the window.

His paws cover his eyes. I rub the golden fur between his ears, but Browny is slow to respond. He whimpers from time to time, as if to complain that he's been lonely without me, he doesn't feel needed, and such is a dog's life.

Browny is such a friendly, good-natured companion. Would he attack when an attack is called for? I kind of doubt it. I think it's better that he didn't take part in my rescue. But how can I blame him for pouting? In his place, I would probably pout too.

Meanwhile, Michael places a mug in my hands. It's filled to the rim with delectable dark chocolate hot cocoa. I start to get cozy, taking in the rich aroma, indulging in the smooth, velvety taste that melts in my mouth.

He squats by my side. "Remember our conversation, when you were still stuck in Pirates' Cove, waiting to be airlifted?"

I take a sip, nod. "Told you my middle name is Trouble."

Michael smiles. "Even if it isn't, it should be."

"I work hard to prove it, don't I?"

"You sure do, sweetheart."

"Thank you, love, for saving me."

"Twice."

I touch my nose to his. "Who's counting?"

My cup drained, Michael takes it from my hands and hurries to the kitchen. I rise up, eager for some more hot chocolate. Instead, he carries a huge bouquet of long stem roses in his hand, so huge I can only see his eyes, twinkling over the edge of the petals. Where he got them in the middle of the night is quite beyond me.

"Remember, sweetheart? I told you that when I propose, you'll have absolutely no doubt about my intentions."

"I do."

Lowering himself to one knee in the most chivalrous manner, Michael hands me the roses and, with great flair, opens a small box where a diamond ring is nestled. Its facets are glinting, taking in the candlelight and reflecting it back.

Just to see how he'll react, I do what I think he least expects. I fall to one knee before him and, before he can say a word, brush a stray curl away from his forehead. Then I whisper, "Michael Morse, will you marry me?"

His eyes shine. "Oh, Ash, I thought you'd never ask!"

"Well?"

"Yes, with all my heart."

✴

I'm so happy, so excited about us—until Michael says, "Let's call your Ma. She should be the first to hear the news."

"At this hour?"

"Why not?"

"Because."

"Because what?"

"Because," I say, grasping for some excuse, "I don't have my cellphone. It was taken by the gang."

"So?" Michael shrugs. "Here's mine."

I hesitate, and he says, "Tell you what: I'll call her."

"No!" I cry. "Hearing a man's voice in an unexpected call, well after midnight, will make her scramble through her usual options, none of them good."

"Such as?"

"Such as," I say, then change my voice to resemble hers. "'Oh my, is this about Ashley? Has she been involved in a car wreck? Is she stranded? Or in the hospital? Shall I come pick her up?'"

Michael laughs heartily, so I try again to make him understand the gravity of what he's about to do. "That's only the beginning," I say. "She'll come up with something even more horrible."

"What can be worse than that?"

"Who knows?" I mimic her again. "'Has Ashley been kidnapped? For ransom? By a crazy person who wants to keep her?'"

Michael gives me a naughty look and places the call before I can stop him. "Crazy I sure am," he says. "About you."

"That's the last thing Ma wants to hear." I listen nervously to the incessant ringing, hoping it'll die down before waking her. "She doesn't much like you."

"She has to deal with it sometime," he says. "What better time than tonight?"

Her voice comes up, with a little grunt.

"Oh no," I whisper. "She's going to have a fit!"

Perhaps she's knocked her phone off the nightstand and is now scrambling to pick it up. "Hello?" Ma sounds confused. "Who is this?"

"Michael."

"Oh. Not you again. Where's Ashley?" she demands. Her heart must be beating out of her chest. "Let me talk to her."

After a short scuffle, I yank the phone from his hand. "Ma, I'm sorry."

"Are you okay? Ashley dear, are you okay?"

"What? Yes, Ma. I'm fine. Michael here thought it would be a good idea to call you, which of course, it isn't. Sorry to wake you—"

"You kidding me? I haven't slept all night, thinking of you!"

"Sorry, Ma. Please, go back to bed."

This is when my mother does the one thing she shouldn't. She tells me what not to do. "Don't you tell me you're back to dating *him*."

She may be regretting the words as soon as they're passing her lips, because there's no better way to make me do the exact opposite of what she wants. I can't even help it. It's just me.

"What I am telling you, Ma, is that I've just asked him to marry me."

"It's not funny. You hear me, Ashley? Not funny!"

"Love you too, Ma."

Michael better figure out a way to appease her before we show up on her doorstep.

He grabs the cellphone. "Mrs. Winters?"

She huffs. "Now what?"

"You know, Ash and I were just talking—"

"I don't want to hear any more," she cuts in. "I know you won't believe it, but I'm too tired to argue."

"Sorry to hear it," he says. "Sorry we called you this late."

"Well, you should be!"

"Before you go, just one thing, Mrs. Winters?"

"What's that?"

"Well, you see, we love your challah bread so much—"

"What's not to like?"

"Exactly," he says. "The recipe must be a family secret, passed from one generation to the next, and you must be guarding it fiercely, as well you should, but—"

"Oh." She must be rolling her eyes. "Here comes the *but*."

"We'd love to learn it from you."

"Baking bread takes time, it takes patience," she says. "I don't think you have it in you—"

"Of course," says Michael. "I won't have it any other way."

Ma takes a deep breath. "You sure?"

"Sure I'm sure," he says. "I love cooking."

"You do?"

"Didn't Ash tell you?"

She doesn't answer, perhaps not wanting to admit that given her attitude, I tell her sparingly about him. Instead she says, "I must warn you: we'll have to spend hours until the dough rises —"

"Good," he says. "I'll invite you to my kitchen and have all the ingredients at hand."

"I'll give you a list."

"Can't wait." He steps away from me and lowers his voice, which makes me perk my ears. "Now, don't tell Ash. We'll do it for her birthday, two weeks from now."

And Ma whispers, "Can Ashley hear me?"

"No."

"You sure she likes surprises? I know I don't."

"We'll have to see."

"I guess so," she says, a bit reluctantly.

He turns around to me, smiles. "Baking with you, Mrs. Winters, is long overdue!"

"Well," Ma says, and this time I can't decide if the tone of her voice is sweet or sour, "welcome to the family, Michael."

~ The End ~

About this Book

From USA Today bestselling author Uvi Poznansky comes a gripping suspense thriller:

Her bullet grazed his head, but the leader of a Russian crime organization is still breathing. One way for Vlad to avoid paying the price for his crimes is to play dead; another is to play dying. For Ash, this is not a game. She must learn his secrets. Only one problem: because of the raging pandemic, she must put her plan on hold.

Vlad slips away from the hospital in a body bag, then develops a brazen fraud scheme that will bilk health insurance companies out of millions of dollars. If not caught in time, he will drive victims to suicide, rob Ash of her identity, and slit her throat.

Will Ash manage to stay one step ahead of him and at the same time, protect her loved ones from contagion?

About the Author

Uvi Poznansky is a *USA TODAY* bestselling, award-winning author, poet and artist. "I paint with my pen," she says, "and write with my paintbrush."

Uvi earned her B. A. in Architecture and Town Planning from the Technion in Haifa, Israel. During her studies and in the years immediately following her graduation, she practiced with an innovative Architectural firm, taking part in the design of a large-scale project, *Home for the Soldier*.

Having moved to Troy, N.Y. with her husband and two children, Uvi received a Fellowship grant and a Teaching Assistantship from the Architecture department at Rensselaer Polytechnic Institute. There, she guided teams in a variety of design projects and earned her M.A. in Architecture. Then, taking a sharp turn in her education, she earned her M.S. degree in Computer Science from the University of Michigan.

During the years she spent in advancing her career—first as an architect, and later as a software engineer, software team leader, software manager and a software consultant (with an emphasis on user interface for medical instruments devices)—she wrote and painted constantly. In addition, she taught art appreciation classes.

Her versatile body of work can be seen in two websites: her blog includes thoughts about the creative process, reader reviews, author interviews, excerpts from her novels, voice clips from her audiobooks, poems and short stories. Her art site includes bronze and ceramic sculptures, paper engineering projects, oil and watercolor paintings, charcoal, pen and pencil drawings, and mixed media.

Coma Confidential, Overkill, Overdose, and *Overdue* are novels in the *Ash Suspense Thrillers with a Dash of Romance* series. With each new case, Ash uses grit and intuition to solve the crime.

Virtually Lace is the first volume in a multi-author thriller series, *High-Tech Crime Solvers*, where the authors bring each other's characters into their books.

My Own Voice, The White Piano, The Music of Us, Dancing with Air, and *Marriage before Death* are novels in the *Still Life with Memories* series, a family saga with a love story that develops in the face of hardship and illness over two generations, starting at the 1980's, then harkening back to WWII when Lenny, a soldier, and Natasha, a rising star, first met. These books are also offered in two bundles: *Apart from Love* and *Apart from War*.

Rise to Power, A Peek at Bathsheba, and *The Edge of Revolt* are novels in *The David Chronicles*, telling the story of David as you have never heard it before: from the king himself, telling the unofficial version, the one he never allowed his court scribes to recount. In his mind, history is written to praise the victorious—but at the last stretch of his illustrious life, he feels an irresistible urge to tell the truth. These books are also offered in a trilogy.

In addition, *The David Chronicles* includes six art collections: *Inspired by Art: Fighting Goliath, Inspired by Art: Fall of a Giant, Inspired by Art: Rise to Power, Inspired by Art: A Peek at Bathsheba, Inspired by Art: The Edge of Revolt,* and *Inspired by Art: The Last Concubine.*

A Favorite Son, a new-age twist on an old yarn, is inspired by the biblical story of Jacob and his mother Rebecca, plotting together against the elderly father Isaac, who is lying on his deathbed.

Twisted is a unique collection, laden with shades of mystery. Here, you will come into a dark, strange world, a hyper-reality where nearly everything is firmly rooted in the familiar—except for some quirky detail that twists the yarn.

Home and *Can We Still Love*, Uvi's deeply moving poetry books in tribute of her father, include her poetry and prose as well as translated poems from the pen of her father, the poet, author and artist Zeev Kachel.

Uvi wrote and illustrated two children's books, *Jess and Wiggle* and *Now I Am Paper*. Watch the beautiful animations she created for these books on YouTube: Jess and Wiggle and Now I Am Paper.

About the Cover

The cover depicts Ash as she escapes the fire she set in the LA headquarters of the Russian gang. My art is storytelling. In many thrillers you have the protagonist as a figure seen from the back, running away as if being chased or chasing. By contrast, I show Ash coming towards us, nearly falling into our arms, so we can directly relate to the daring it takes to do what she does in spite of the fear.

I also gave a lot of thought to making each part of this cover shimmer with texture and light, creating an explosive, dynamic urban backdrop for her.

Here is the excerpt describing the scene:

I suck in a deep breath and duck through the flame in search of Mrs. Komarov. I'm guided by her frantic shrieks as a burning beam has collapsed next to her. Her babushka, now removed from her head, is now held with her quivering fingers, covering her mouth and nose from the smoke. We grab her arms and drag her together step by step around the overturned table, across a puddle of spilled Okroshka soup, and out to the street, where an ambulance has just arrived.

We carry her past the cops who surround the place and past the firefighters who are setting up their equipment. The old woman complains, her voice scratchy from smoke inhalation, about the stinging in her eyes.

Medics arrive. They apply medication over the burn on her right side to relieve the pain. They also suggest we get tested for COVID-19.

"Oh no," says Mrs. Komarov. "I heard all about the nasal swab test."

One of the medics explains, "It captures a lot of viral material concentrated in the back of the nose—"

"It is notoriously unpleasant." She coughs. "You are not going to stick that thing up my nose!"

"No worries. We offer also a saliva test. It's easy. All you have to do is spit into a sterilized container, which is then sent to the lab for processing. The results will be available in a few hours."

"Fine. Spitting I like."

Strangely, the one person missing through all of this is her son. For a second, I think I see him across the street, watching us. A sudden rush of adrenaline sends me dashing over there, ready to point him out for the cops—only to realize there's no one there. What I saw must have been a phantom of imagination, a dance of flames.

Acknowledgments

I would like to give recognition to four authors who read this book while it was still in a half-cooked state and with great generosity, offered their comments, insights and suggestions. I am deeply grateful to them.

S.R. Mallery, two-time Readers' Favorite Gold Medal Winner, is the author of Tea, Anyone (cozy mystery), Sewing Can be Dangerous, The Dolan Girls, Unexpected Gifts, Tales to Count On, and Trouble in Glamour Town. She weaves historical fiction into her stories with a delicate thread.

Sheila Deeth, a high-ranking book reviewer and an editor, has a Bachelors and Masters in mathematics from Cambridge University, England. She is the author of Exodus Tales, Bethlehem Baby, Divide by Zero, and Infinite Sum.

Aaron Paul Lazar is a multi-award winning mystery author. He created the Gus LeGarde mystery series (featuring protagonist Gus LeGarde, a classical music professor.)

Paul Douglas Lovell is the author of autobiographical stories, including Playing Out, Paulyanna, and Empty Corridors.

A Note to the Reader

Thank you for reading this book! If you enjoyed it, I invite you to check out more books from the same pen. There is always a new project on my drawing board, so please come back to check it out.

I would love to hear what you thought of this book. You have the power of bringing it to the attention of more readers, by posting your own review. It would mean so much to me.

And another thing you can do to help me spread the word is this: please tell your friends about my work. How else will they hear about the story? How else will the characters, who sprang from my mind onto these pages, leap from there into new minds?

Bonus Excerpts
Excerpt: Coma Confidential

Rhythms of footfalls are intensifying outside my hospital room. It must be morning. Immobile, all I can do is count beats. I must have spent days here—who knows, maybe even weeks—or else I wouldn't be able to tell time by means of listening to echoes.

It's a new skill, a new gain for me, barely significant enough to offset the loss of something far more important: my identity. Even so, I'm proud. I pat myself on the back. Mentally.

By their patter, I know that two pair of shoes have just stepped into the room. It doesn't take much to figure who is standing in them. The two nurses prattle about having to change my feeding tube. In a blink, a craving comes over me.

Oh, what I would give for a decent donut! I drool at the thought of dunking it into a bowl filled with smooth, warm, vanilla-flavored sugar glaze, then lifting it to my mouth for a quick lick.

One of the nurses wipes the dribble off my chin. I wish she would stop handling me. I wish I could turn my head away.

Meanwhile, my stomach is growling. I'm so hungry. At this point, never mind pastry. I'll take any real food—even peas and carrots, which normally I hate. Being able to chew them would cast me back among the living.

In this sorry state, I've come to acquire a new affinity with vegetables. Maybe they have feelings, too. Maybe they dread being poked about with a fork, just as much as I fear being injected. Maybe being sucked down that dark, cavernous windpipe to be consumed by something yet unknown is repulsive to them. I think that at long last, I understand carrots and peas. So no, I'm never going to put them in my mouth again.

Seriously, I prefer donuts.

"Oh my! Accident?" asks one nurse, while pumping liquid food into my stomach with a syringe.

"No, worse than that," says the other one. By comparison, her voice is lower and more mature. It is also secretive.

"What can be worse than an accident?"

"Don't even ask."

"Fine, then. Let's talk about something else."

"Like what?"

"Like, what d'you want to be, ten years from now?"

There's a faint sound—maybe the older nurse is scratching her head—which leaves the question unanswered. Oh, the things I'd say, if only I could revive my vocal cords! I'd shout, "Ten years, are you kidding me? Who cares! I just want to make it through today!"

But on second thought, I want more than that, much more. I strain my vocal cords in a desperate attempt to cry out, "I want to wake up from this nightmare, at the snap of my fingers. I want to walk away from this bed. Most of all, I want to know who I am. Is that too much to ask?"

Excerpt: Overkill

Ed lies still on the sidewalk, his eyelids open but unflinching. The only thing about him that moves are the lapels of his corduroy coat, flapping slightly this way and that across his neck as the wind floats chilly feelers over his body.

Timmy gasps—but his eyes are not tearful, not yet. In that second, when time slows, the driver side door is swaying with an annoying noise. With each squeak, the child takes a gulp of air as if about to ask, "Dad, will you get up? Will you grab the door handle?"

No blood is visible, at first. So, I too allow myself to wonder: Will Ed climb back into his seat, dust off his shoulders, and wave goodbye to his son, before driving away?

I expect him to do so. Almost.

Until another round of gunshots blasts the air.

Without even thinking, I push Timmy down to the asphalt, which is quite easy because he's such a skinny child and utterly in shock. Then I land hard on my elbows beside him and push a hand against his chest until he crawls backwards, until he butts against his father's car. It casts a shadow over him. At the moment, there is no better place to hide.

Up on the pavement, a short distance from us, blood starts puddling around Ed's shoulder. I try to block Timmy from seeing it.

He shakes his head, still in disbelief.

Please, God, no. This can't be true.

Everything around us is in a state of utter confusion. The sidewalk is strewn with abandoned backpacks, as some pupils are running for their lives. Others cower behind a bush or a car. One uses his flimsy umbrella as a shield.

A teacher cries out to him, "Duck!"

And another teacher, by the gate of the school, yells, "Run! Get inside! Get down, crawl under your desks! And for Heaven's sake, stay away from the windows!"

A couple of parents attempt getting out of their cars to pull their children to safety, but at the sound of shooting they drop to their knees with empty arms.

Next to me, Timmy turns onto his stomach, mashes his nose against the tire, and wedges himself, somehow, between the curb and the Ford. Then he crawls under it toward the rear bumper, making room for me, too.

I try to cock my head up from the damp surface. Looking at the scene from under the belly of a car is a whole different experience. Someone stands at the other side of the car, and all I can see is his sneakers, socks, and the hem of his coat, flaring at its bottom. Also, the muzzle of his gun. For a heartbeat, before dark clouds close in, it glints in the sunlight.

I reach over and clamp a hand over Timmy's mouth to prevent him from screaming, from drawing the killer's attention. A hail of bullets rains down, sparking off the front bumper.

Timmy tenses up. His breath trembles as it escapes my touch. I must protect him. I must bring him back safely to his mother.

The edge of the curb gouges into my back. I adjust, I turn over. Now it presses against my belly.

I must not lose this child, either.

Now, the killer kicks the grill of the car, then jams his weapon, hard, into the front window. I know it by seeing only one of his feet on the ground and by the sound of cracking. It reverberates all over as the car shakes. Shards of glass come pinging against the asphalt and stab at my fingers.

Why is he wasting his time—at the risk of being identified, or even caught—on an empty car, when all around us, juicier targets come into his view?

Excerpt: Overdose

Perched on the exam table, I'm desperately searching for a way out. There isn't any.

Even worse: I've drained my energy trying to resist him, with little to show other than a long scratch across the wall as he carried me to this room. Exhausted, I have no breath left in me.

In a blink, my entire life passes before me. Pa always wished for me to make my mark. Have I?

Not if Kabir is about to blot it out.

He sets the wine flask on a nearby desk, using his elbow to shove some medical instruments out of the way. Maybe because of some force of habit, Kabir takes a piece of clothing—green medical scrubs, of all things—off a hook on the door, and puts it on right over the white polo shirt he's wearing, so the Tommy Hilfiger appliqué on its front pocket is no longer visible. The impostor is now in costume.

Then he pulls open a drawer and takes out a small bottle, filled with pills. I strain my eyes to read the label, but from where I'm sitting, it's a bit too far.

Kabir casts a sly look at me. His lips curl, as if he's about to tell some joke. "This is the single most prescribed psychiatric medication in the U.S. I ought to know, not only because I am a medical professional and not only because I married into a family that owns a pharmaceutical company but also because of my wife. She passed away because of it. Overdose, you know."

Kabir takes a pause, perhaps to see if I would ask anything about her death. I don't. Why upset him? What's at risk at this point is my own life!

A moment later, he pivots to an entirely different subject. In his professional tone, he asks, "Are you pregnant, or plan to become pregnant?"

"Not anytime soon!" I gasp, somewhat in shock. "Why?"

"Because." He shakes the bottle to a loud rattle. "Your pills are about to run out."

"Pills? What pills?"

"Xanax."

He steps closer to me and raises the bottle to my unbelieving eyes. The name, printed on the label in bold letters, is mine.

"What? That can't be!" I cry. "I'm not on any medication, let alone this—"

"You've been taking it for months, to treat your anxiety."

"Oh no, I haven't—"

"Why try to deny it?" Kabir laughs in my face. "You seem to be in panic, even now!"

About that, he's right. But the only cure for my dread is for him to let me go, which is doubtful, or for me to find a way around him, which is far-fetched.

Kabir crushes a bunch of pills into a small heap of powder, transfers it to a glass, and pours some wine into it, all in plain view, as if wanting to show me the method of my own demise.

I can't afford to give him what he seems to want: the pleasure of seeing how scared I am.

He swirls the wine about, then raises it to my nose, so I may smell its aroma. "I'm happy to hear you're not expecting a baby." His tone is loaded with sarcasm. "I wouldn't want it to suffer any ill-effects, once you have your little drink."

I brace myself into being stubborn. "You can't force me."

"You know I can." He coughs up a sharp laugh. "And then, there would be no more need to have this prescription renewed."

What I want—even more than a chance to save myself—is to give the doctor a taste of his own medicine.

In a heartbeat, my hands turn clammy. "I don't know what I did to deserve this."

He growls, "Sure you do! You've been asking too many questions about me, about my trip to India years ago, and about the woman I married there. No one gets to do all that and live to tell the tale."

I hesitate to ask, "Not even your wife?"

"Especially not her."

"What about me?" I ask, already knowing the answer. "Am I going to survive the night?"

"Trust me, it is with a heavy heart that I must kill you." Kabir comes closer, strokes my chin. "Such a beauty." For a second, his eyes seem sad, almost. "Such a waste."

Excerpt: Virtually Lace

Even before Michael spotted the body, the idea of creating a simulation of the scene occurred to him. At sunset, the panoramic view of Laguna Beach was awe-inspiring. He wondered if he could render it convincingly in his model, the virtual reality model which he had been developing in the back of his garage for months, until the recent acquisition of his software by a military ops company.

Could beauty be taken apart without loss of emotional impact? Could its data be synthesized, somehow, into a lifelike experience? In short, could he apply his analytical skills to fool his own senses?

For now, these were purely academic questions. They occupied his mind, which helped him forget his loneliness. Michael brought his car to a stop at the corner of Cliff Drive and let it maneuver by itself into a tight parking spot. In all probability, this evening would be uneventful, or so he thought. It was the end of April. He had nothing to do and no one to do it with.

Sitting there awhile, lost in his thoughts, how was he to know that in the coming days he was going to revisit this place, starting at this particular intersection, to examine every possible angle, every conceivable point of view?

The shadow of the lamppost grew longer. It prowled over to the pavement on the other side, where it lost its sharpness. The evening breeze turned overhead with a shriek, only to fall into a whoosh. Michael imagined it whispering, of all things, of murder at dusk. What a crazy idea! Where did that come from?

At 8:03pm came the sound of footfalls. A teenage girl was walking down the street so fast that the uneven click of her heels was already passing him by, leaving a faint whiff of perfume. No, that must have been some other fragrance, perhaps the saltiness of the sea, drifting over the sweetness of creek milkweeds and Belladonna lilies.

Where had he seen her before?

By the time he got out of the car, the girl had already crossed to the other side. With each step, the white dress whipped across her legs and fluttered, fold upon fold, in the cold wind.

His soles beat an echo in the empty street. He didn't mind the occasional squeak, because he had just bought them.

Electric lights buzzed in the buildings behind him, and foxtail ferns hissed, swaying along the trail. Her shadow flitted over the shrubs, falling farther and farther out of reach.

Before reaching the bend, she glanced over her shoulder and for a heartbeat, met his eyes. In some ways she reminded him of his ex-girlfriend, Ash, whom he hadn't seen since the *incident*. What was it that drew him to this girl? Why was he looking, time and again, to save a damsel in distress?

There was a certain quality about that look, which he couldn't put into words. Anguish? No, it was more acute than that. The closest he could name it was fear.

Excerpt: Marriage before Death

Without uttering a sound I gave her a look, begging her to leave. Rochelle gave one to me, begging me to play along.

Out loud she said, "Oh how I hate you! I hate you now more than I ever loved you!"

At that, the SS officer burst out laughing. It lasted quite a while, or so it seemed to me, and by the time it finally ended, a cruel smile was left across his face, stretching from one pointy ear to the other.

"*Ach*," he hissed. "What a woman! Cold one minute—hot the next!"

Rochelle hung her eyes on me one more time.

"At the very least," she implored, "you should say you are sorry, so sorry to have left me in such a difficult situation!"

The SS officer cut in.

"Didn't I tell you?" he asked her. "His kind, they have no morals! Worse than animals is what they are."

She turned away and went back to his side. From there she said, in a tone of regret, "Right you are. I was naive, up to now, to hope for anything different from him."

Over her sorrow, the SS officer went on to say, "How could you ever let yourself be seduced by such a man?"

She shook her head. "How silly of me! How foolish it is to hope! I was sure he would confirm to everyone here his desire to marry me."

To which the SS officer said, "Now, mademoiselle, you have learned your lesson."

She gave him a tearful smile, but then could not help crying out to me, "Oh, for heaven's sake, don't you get it? I'm expecting your child!"

At that I had a change of heart. Why? First, because I was moved to tears by her plea, no matter if it was a fake one or not; and second, because what had I got to lose?

So I uttered, "Forgive me, Rochelle."

"What?" she asked. "What did you say?"

"Forgive me," I said, with a catch in my throat. "If I were a free man I would gladly keep my promise to you."

A triumphant smile played on her red lips. Yet, for just a moment, she was silent.

I thought she might make peace with me, now that I relented. Instead, she turned to the SS officer.

"Herr Müller," she said. "I'm not here to beg for mercy for this man."

In surprise, "You're not?" he asked, raising a thick eyebrow.

And from the other side of the table, his French collaborator echoed, "You're not?"

My face was still burning, still stinging from that slap of hers. I bit my lips to overcome the pain. If I could muster the nerve to speak up once more, I would ask her the very same thing.

Really? You're not?

"No," she stressed.

The toothbrush mustache under Herr Müller's nose started to twitch. Perhaps he was becoming suspicious of her.

"I thought," he said, "that you had a big favor to ask of me."

And she said, "I do."

And he said, "Well? What is it, then?"

"For the sake of my family," said Rochelle, "for the pride of my father, for my own honor, and for the future of this baby, I cannot be an unwed mother! I'd rather die!"

Becoming somewhat impatient, "*Ach!*" he said. "You should have thought of that earlier, before you got involved with the likes of him."

It was then that she said, "I promise, Herr Müller, giving me what I ask for is sure to give you the greatest pleasure, because it is just what this man deserves."

"Which is what?"

"Marriage before death."

Books by Uviart

Coma Confidential

(Volume I of *Ash Suspense Thrillers with a Dash of Romance*)

Kindle: B07L92YHST Paperback: 978-1791691592

Overkill

(Volume II of *Ash Suspense Thrillers with a Dash of Romance*)

Kindle: B084GDK156 Paperback: 979-8644328192

Overdose

(Volume III of *Ash Suspense Thrillers with a Dash of Romance*)

Kindle: B07VP4S6PK Paperback: 978-1086703665

Overdue

(Volume IV of *Ash Suspense Thrillers with a Dash of Romance*)

Kindle: B08S724T4G Paperback: 979-8599499671

Ash Suspense Thrillers: Trilogy

(Volume I-III of *Ash Suspense Thrillers with a Dash of Romance*)

Kindle: B0893MJNSY Paperback: 979-8648269644

Virtually Lace

(Volume I of *High-Tech Crime Solvers*)

Kindle: B07L968RXD Paperback: 978-1790407187

My Own Voice

(Volume I of *Still Life with Memories*)

Kindle: B013TA3FBS Paperback: 978-0984993215

The White Piano

(Volume II of *Still Life with Memories*)

Kindle: B013TAU7L4 Paperback: 978-1517049447

The Music of Us

(Volume III of *Still Life with Memories*)

Kindle: B013TCYWHC Paperback: 978-0-9849932-9-1

Dancing with Air

(Volume IV of *Still Life with Memories*)
Kindle: B01I4ENROY Paperback: 978-1536896534

Marriage before Death

(Volume V of *Still Life with Memories*)
Kindle: B0746NW5CD Paperback: 978-1974001736

Apart from Love

(*Still Life with Memories Bundle I*)
Kindle: B006WPITP0 Paperback: 978-0-9849932-0-8

Apart from War

(*Still Life with Memories Bundle II*)
Kindle: B07MMZLD7Z Paperback: 978-1792131592

Rise to Power
(Volume I of *The David Chronicles*)
Kindle: B00H6PMZ0U Paperback: 978-0-9849932-4-6

A Peek at Bathsheba
(Volume II of *The David Chronicles*)
Kindle: B00LEPPDV6 Paperback: 978-0-9849932-7-7

The Edge of Revolt
(Volume III of *The David Chronicles*)
Kindle: B00Q5WVKA6 Paperback: 978-0984993284

The David Chronicles: Trilogy
(Volume I-III of *The David Chronicles*)
Kindle: B00QYGF6WG Paperback: 978-1797440699

The David Chronicles: Art
(Volume IV-XI of *The David Chronicles*)
Kindle: B08YWSH7HC Paperback: 979-8721612886

Inspired by Art: Fighting Goliath

(Art book. Volume IV of *The David Chronicles*)

Kindle: B01MSBNSE4   Paperback 978-1797726212

Inspired by Art: Fall of a Giant

(Art book. Volume V of *The David Chronicles*)

Kindle: B01MSBS82Q   Paperback: 978-1092307765

Inspired by Art: Rise to Power

(Art book. Volume VI of *The David Chronicles*)

Kindle: B01N2786VX   Paperback: 978-1092263207

Inspired by Art: A Peek at Bathsheba

(Art book. Volume VII of *The David Chronicles*)

Kindle: B01MUFS9OA   Paperback: 978-1092306225

Inspired by Art: The Edge of Revolt

(Art book. Volume VIII of *The David Chronicles*)

Kindle: B01N6ZG0W8   Paperback: 978-1091306158

Inspired by Art: The Last Concubine

(Art book. Volume IX of *The David Chronicles*)

Kindle: B01N2AXQP2   Paperback: 978-1092302715

A Favorite Son

Kindle: B00AUZ3LGU Paperback: 978-0-9849932-5-3

Twisted

Kindle: B00D7Q3IY4

Paperback: 978-0984993260 Nook: 2940151689588

Home

(Poetry)

Kindle: B00960TE3Y

Paperback: 978-09849932-3-9 Nook: 2940151729468

Can We Still Love

(Poetry)

Kindle: B0GV3G23V4 Paperback: B0GY8Q1Y9Z

Virtually Yummy: Recipes that Inspire

(Cookbook)

Kindle: B085BDNDM5 Nook: 2940163988655

Apple: id1501182051 Kobo: 9781393589853

בית

(Poetry in Hebrew)
Paperback: 978-1494920968
Apple: id1302908918 Kobo: 9781540199966

Jess and Wiggle

Kindle: B013D1W0SM Paperback: 978-1494920968

Now I Am Paper

Kindle: B00YQS4O72 Paperback: 978-1494919429